Plague In Our Midst

by **Gregg Albers, MD.**

HUNTINGTON HOUSE, INC.
P.O. Box 53788 Lafayette, Louisiana 70505

Copyright © 1988 by **Gregg Albers**

All rights reserved. No part of this book may be reproduced without permission from the publisher, except by a reviewer who may quote brief passages in a review; nor may any part of this book be reproduced, stored in a retrieval system or copied by mechanical, photocopying, recording or other means, without permission from the publisher.

Huntington House, Inc.
P.O. Box 53788, Lafayette, Louisiana 70505

Library of Congress Catalog Card Number 88-081729
ISBN Number 0-910311-51-X

Cover design and typography by Publications Technologies
Printed by Faith Press Intl. Inc., Tyler, Texas

TABLE OF CONTENTS

Foreword 5
  1. The Church in a Sexual World 7
  2. The Plague of Aids 25
  3. The Biblical Perspective of Sexuality 39
  4. The World's Sexuality 51
  5. Sex Education and Scriptural Principles 63
  6. Teaching Children About Sexual Attitudes 77
  7. Adolescent Sexual Attitudes 97
  8. Sexual Maturation and Function 119
  9. Sexual Problems and Issues 139
 10. Design for Revival 161
Epilogue 173

FOREWORD

There are several explosive issues facing today's teenagers, among them sexuality and other related problems. Families have been influenced by humanism, secularism, and unchecked sexual abuse through entertainment and news from media sources. Now we are paying the price in AIDS, teenage pregnancies, and a number of other sexual diseases. Many young people are not able to talk with their parents about these problems. Also, peer pressure to have sex drives young people further into these dangers. Being a Christian does not solve these problems because approximately 60 percent of Christian young people are giving into these pressures and having sexual intercourse before marriage.

Just as there is no one source for the problem, there is no one solution. Dr. Gregg Albers suggests that communication between Christian young people and their parents is one of the answers. Young people need instruction and role models, but most importantly, they need an adult with whom they can share their joys, sorrows, triumphs, and problems. Teens want to find "love" through sex, but physical sex never substitutes for true love. Young people need to base their love in a relationship with their parents first, then branch out through biblical principles to love their mate and life partner.

The problem of sex has been complicated by AIDS. One sexual mistake can destroy a life. This is more than losing virginity or destroying one's morality. One mistake can kill a person in two to five years. According to Surgeon General Everett Koop, the only way to stop AIDS is through sexual abstinence and to say "no" to illegal drugs. Even though the message, "Say 'no' to drugs" is emphasised in the media, it must become a reality in the life of young people. Parents need to understand this danger and communicate it to their children.

Dr. Albers points out that the plague is not just AIDS. It is sexuality gone rampant in America. He is not just a wild-eyed prophet who is announcing the judgment of AIDS against America. He is a medical doctor who has written a book to wake up parents to the task of communicating sexuality to their children. The solution is not just medical tests or coming up with a medical solution to AIDS. The solution is returning to the traditional family values that were taught in the American home and a return to communication between parents and children. These values have arisen out of our Christian ethic which is based in the Word of God.

—*Dr. Elmer L. Towns.*

Dr. Towns is the author of more than 50 books with total sales of more than one million copies. Three of these are listed on the Christian Booksellers List of Bestsellers. He is a noted seminar speaker, founder of the Church Growth Institute, Vice President of Liberty University and Dean of the B.R. Lakin School of Religion.'

CHAPTER ONE
The Church in a Sexual World

I can still remember the numb sensation when I hung up the telephone — that sickening heaviness compressing my head, my chest, making my arms and legs feel like lead. It was a phone call from a Christian brother and a dear friend that jolted me into the reality of a sexual world.

Jay had been my friend for 15 years. We had met soon after I was saved at Miami University. He always had such a warm, caring attitude for others, a genuine Christlikeness. He was selfless, always thinking of others' needs. All that mattered to him was the spiritual condition, the joy of others.

Ministry was in his heart. He often helped at a large inner-city mission, counseling and praying with the down-and-outers. It was his compassion and love for others that led him to Haiti, to minister through a school construction project in 1979.

My friend had called me for some medical counsel and help. A few months before he was admitted to a local hospital for bleeding somewhere in the intestines. Test after test was run to find out why his platelet count had dropped so low. The bleeding continued; platelet transfusions were not helping.

Jay's doctors decided to remove his spleen, the organ that appeared to be "soaking-up" these miniscule clotting factors. But the cause for this mysterious ailment remained elusive until one resident physician decided to run an AIDS test. The resident had seen a similar case described in a journal.

When the physician attending Jay entered the room, he started to ask some very strange questions.

"Have you ever taken intravenous drugs, had a homosexual affair or intercourse, or had sex with a prostitute?"

Jay was deeply offended by these questions and knew that something extremely serious had been discovered in one of the tests.

With tears in his eyes, he asked "What kind of disease do I have?"

"You have AIDS, a very serious disorder of your immune system."

Jay had never received a transfusion, never had intercourse and never used intravenous drugs. But he had contracted AIDS.

Later, when he was able to talk again with the physician he gave him a thorough history of his travel to foreign countries. The missions trip to Haiti in 1979 was complicated by an illness, where Jay had to run from bed to bathroom for two days straight. A local dispensary had given him and three other high school students who were traveling with the team injections for the diarrhea and nausea. The needle was wiped with alcohol, when that was available, and reused on many different patients.

His compassion, his loving heart to serve others and his

Plague in Our Midst

desire to serve God had led Jay to Haiti, the place where he was infected with AIDS.

"Will I be able to get married? What are all these infections the doctors are saying I'll contract? Is there any cure for AIDS? Are there ways I can keep myself healthier through nutrition and exercise? Am I going to die from this thing?"

As I listened to the desperation in his voice, I kept asking myself, "Why Jay? Why someone so innocent?"

Attempting to put aside my feelings for this Christian brother, trying to put on my most professional sounding demeanor, I answered Jay's questions slowly and with as much unemotional information as I could muster. Never before had I discussed imminent death with such a young patient in my years of medical practice, especially one whom I knew so well, one I loved so much as a brother, one who was so innocent.

My prayer time that night was impossible. All I could do was to think about Jay, about that clinic in Haiti, about the pain and suffering that would follow. Tears welled up in my eyes as I remembered the encouragement we had once shared in Bible study, the prayers we had spoken for each other's needs. All that mentally materialized were the inconsistencies — a deadly venereal disease striking someone who had never been sexually active, a saint dying of a disease of decadence and uncontrolled lust.

Then my mind quickly raced to my own children and my wife. Could AIDS affect the ones I love, the family that I daily lift to God's throne for protection and health? Could my precious little girls or my strong-willed boys ever be afflicted with a disease that has spread through homosexual promiscuity, through intravenous drug addiction? How could I defend those who look to me for wisdom, nurture and protection from this plague?

My sleep that night was restless, to say the least.

One cool, spring afternoon about a month after I had heard about Jay's dilemma, I read a newspaper and was shocked by the news of "Scandal in the Church." Almost every newspaper in America had carried the lead story: "Evangelist Admits to Sexual Tryst With Church Secretary."

As a physician I often hear about strange and sordid situations and, to be honest, am often not shocked by many of the things that I see or hear. But I remember being stunned, not by the situation, but by the person involved. How could a man, so loved and trusted by other believers, so effective through his ministry, become involved in such immoral behavior?

Soon the story became even more perverse. Charges of homosexual advances and gestures, financial mismanagement, payoffs for silence and huge salaries for "favorites" broke into the news. Counter-charges of "ministry stealing," lying, misrepresentation and dramatic scheming filled the papers until a "holy war" was raging out of control. The credibility of many Christian ministries was shattered by these events. The gospel became a derision; believers were mocked; ministries lost their financial base for operations leading to huge cutbacks in personnel and budgets.

The stature of fundamental Christianity had sustained severe damage, both through the sin itself and through the lack of repentance by the individuals involved. They displayed only self-righteousness when explaining their financial sins. The only things that mattered to them were "forgiveness" and the clearing of their names so that they could return quickly to the spotlight.

Again that nauseating numbness gripped me as I pondered the possible fallout from this scandal, the credibility destroyed, the money wasted and the pain of the victims. My mind flashed back to the situation with Jay, where others' sexual promiscuity caused his pain and imminent death. The church was in great pain and suffering as well because of the sexual immorality of a few.

And then it struck again. A full year had not elapsed before the second major scandal hit the church. Another

Plague in Our Midst

well-known television preacher had admitted his addiction to pornographic acts that were viewed in person, not by video or film. A picture of this minister entering a motel with a known prostitute broke into the headlines and all he could do was tearfully admit his sin to his church, his family and his multi-national audience and step down from the pulpit.

At least his repentance appeared genuine.

What would these scandals, and the sexual indiscretions still to be unveiled, mean to the church? Had sexual promiscuity become a serious problem within the church, our last bastion of spiritual safety in a sinful world? Will this sexual promiscuity lead to church members becoming infected with AIDS and potentially spreading it to other believers? What about the youth within the church and reports of premarital intercourse in 60-80 percent of these young persons? What is the church's responsibility in preaching against sexual sin, and how can the message be relayed to promiscuous individuals both inside and outside of the church? Is promiscuity within the church receiving God's chastisement through the AIDS epidemic as the Jews received plagues because of their sinful rebellion?

Question after question raced through my mind until reality again struck at my heart. What did this problem of sexuality in the church mean to my family?

The resemblance between Jay's situation and the church, the virgin bride of Christ, was uncanny. Just as Jay had contracted a disease of decadence through a needle, so the innocent and unsuspecting church has been injected with the world's sickness, sin sickness. Both are sick, both appear to be badly infected.

There appears to be no way of hiding from promiscuity in the church or from the spread of AIDS except by seeking God's grace and deliverance. He allows trials to arise in the lives of believers, problems that seem to defy solution. We attempt to hide from these problems. We devise man-made programs to divert our attention. But only through direct obedience to God's Word and through trust in His protection can we grow through adverse trials and testings.

There was no place left to turn for answers as I envisioned this double plague of uncontrollable disease and debauchery within the church. There was no place except to seek God's help, guidance, strength and grace.

Again, reality had struck home.

THE NEED TO KNOW

My prayful concern is for my family and for my extended family in Christ. What can we do to protect ourselves, the ones we love, from the spread of this deadly, rapidly disseminating disease? Through the study of God's Word, some very simple and essential information becomes apparent. Violation of the Word of God will bring sin-sickness and physical disease to the person and to the society that condones such behaviors. Obedience to these principles brings God's promise of protection and blessing.

Families, God's ordained unit of nurturing, love-giving and values-education must be encouraged to teach children about the biblical principles governing proper sexual attitudes and function. I, as a father, must teach my children to obey all of God's Word, especially the teachings about sexuality. Then God's protection and blessing will abound in my family as together we obey Him.

It also became evident that, as a Christian physician, I had a strong moral and spiritual duty to teach my patients about the dangers of AIDS through understanding God's principles and through obedience.

In my years of practice, I have dealt with scores of sexual disasters within Christian homes — fathers who have had incestuous relations with their daughters and daughters who must live with the pain of this "dirty secret;" families that were destroyed by the promiscuity of the father or mother, by adultery leading to divorce; pastors or church helpers who desired sex with children, often because of previous sexual abuse by a pedophile when they were young; teen women who attempted suicide or sought abortion because of an unplanned pregnancy; mothers who are

Plague in Our Midst

raped and beaten by their own husbands; the destruction of a marriage over the use of pornography; a woman and her newborn child both dying of AIDS because of the husband's "need" for a prostitute.

This book is written out of compassion for these families — families just like yours and mine — and out of a desire to protect my patients — my brothers and sisters — who are tempted to sexual sin. My family needs the information in this book just as your family does, to awaken us to this difficult reality and to protect us from the plague in our midst.

PROMISCUITY IN THE CHURCH

It took the "scandal" in Charlotte N.C., to fully awaken me to the reality of promiscuous sexuality in the church. I just did not want to admit that it was that serious a problem. Some recent studies on Christian teen promiscuity completed by leading experts in the field had shown that most, between 60-80 percent of young people, have had sexual intercourse prior to marriage. This is about the same as non-Christian teens. There is no doubt that it is a serious problem.

And the solution, family education, is similarly in very serious trouble. Only 20-25 percent of parents ever talk to their children about sexuality, and even fewer talk with their children or teens about the biblical principles of sexuality. This too is similar to secular studies where only 20 percent of adults talked with their children about sexual attitudes or function. These statistics terrify me because I know, personally, how difficult it is to change human behavior through education.

The scandal in Charlotte has allowed many of us to see and believe that sexual promiscuity within the church is a serious problem that must be confronted. I am always saddened when I hear of an adulterous situation leading to divorce, sexual abuse or incest in the home or the contracting of some venereal disease through disobedience. It always seems much harder to understand and deal with when it is a Christian family that is affected.

The personal devastation that is wrought by an unquenchable desire to fulfill a sinful, sexual temptation continues to be appalling. I am aware of and have counseled many. These situations that you will read about here, just as the story about Jay, are true; but the names, places and circumstances have been changed to protect the identities of these dear believers. The pain and devastation is equally true, and much more vivid when experienced in person.

When he first arrived in the small Pennsylvania town, where he had been called to pastor a small, dynamic Baptist church, John was greatly admired. He was tall, with dark flowing hair, and a beautifully resonant bass voice. His fire and enthusiasm for witness, for building a strong local body of believers, easily identified him as the new spiritual leader.
But after many years of stress and extremely long hours of selfless ministry to others, his marriage started to crumble. His wife could not bear the long hours of separation and became an emotional wreck. She sought help from one counselor after another. In the midst of this turmoil, possibly as a result, a sexual affair with the church secretary occurred. This sexual relationship continued for years.
Within months, many persons were dismayed at how things were changing. Church attendance started to drop as John's sermons lacked the special anointing of the Holy Spirit. Members started to leave; financial problems ensued.
Some faithful men and deacons in the church confronted Pastor John with his now "well-known" sin; but his unrepentant heart and his legal manipulation of church bylaws to prevent his withdrawal shocked these men of God into open weeping. They were powerless to do anything except leave the ministry they loved, the ministry in which their lives were invested. No longer did love exist between this pastor and his flock.

Jenny was a beautiful, blonde-headed, west-coast girl who grew up in a strong Christian family. She loved to hear

Plague in Our Midst

Bible stories at bedtime, especially when her father would read from the children's Bible book. She loved her father and would do anything to please him. Friends could see the perfection of their relationship in Jenny's younger days.

But as she grew, their relationship drew apart. They no longer spent the quality time together they had years earlier. Duties of job and church placed a heavy burden on her father's shoulders. Friends could see the strain between the two, almost a fearful spirit when Jenny's father approached her.

The first time I met Jenny was in my office. She sulked across the room, her gaze on the floor, and fell heavily into a folding chair. Her face appeared sullen and depressed. There was little eye contact when we talked. She was complaining of severe stomach cramps and occasional vomiting. When I asked how things were going with school, family and friends, she just whispered, "Fine."

"You look a little depressed today. Is there something that you would like to talk about?" I asked.

"I just came here for some medication, not a sermon!" she snapped back in anger.

The second time I saw Jenny was in the emergency room. She had an I.V. in each arm, a tube in her nose and mouth and a breathing machine that was pushing air into her almost lifeless body. She had taken an overdose of Valium, her mother's medication.

Two days later, the tube was removed and she could speak. I took the opportunity to ask again if she wanted to talk about something, but she just turned the other way. I had not yet earned her trust.

I heard what happened later from a female mental health worker who had the chance to talk with her about the overdose. Jenny had begun to talk about the problems she was having at home. Over the next few days, the whole, sad story unfolded.

She had been sexually molested by her father many times over a couple of years. She had been beaten, raped and threatened that, if she would ever tell, worse would happen. In the midst of her guilt, she had sex with five boys, usually older than she. At the age of 14, she was pregnant and her father, fearing the child was his, forced her to have an abortion. She had been unable emotionally to handle the pain and suffering and on two other occasions had taken her mother's Valium, trying to end her nightmare.

I have ministered to scores of these victims of the "new age of sexual freedom," the persons who are in bondage to their own lusts and desires, the families that are shattered with the immorality of a loved and trusted member. The effect of sinfulness chain-reacts to a society that is reaping the diseases and plagues of sexual debauchery. Sexuality has defiled a church whose witness and members are tarnished, whose ministry is diminished in stature.

Could these problems — adultery, incest, sexual abuse, teen pregnancy — occur in your family or mine? Without a willingness to admit that this serious problem exists and without the motivation to obey God's directions, our families are at risk. Without the essential information about promiscuity, members of our family may be enticed to make that one fatal, sexual mistake. From the positive standpoint, if we are willing to face this situation with prayer and education, we will be motivated to obey these scriptural principles, bringing God's protection and blessing to our loved ones.

ISSUES OF SEXUALITY

If you want to be aware of the sad reality of sexual promiscuity in our world, then you should spend time in a large-city emergency room. The years I spent there during my medical training allowed me to see the full array of the world's decadence.

I remember one morning, at 3 a.m., sprinting down the corridor to attend our third gunshot patient of the evening. The first young man, black, 20 years old, was shot three

Plague in Our Midst

times in the chest by his girlfriend, because he had admitted to having another regular sex partner. He died.

The second episode was even more twisted. One customer of a well known prostitute was slashed with an "emergency room scalpel," stolen at her last visit. He had not payed her lofty $150 fee. She didn't like it and filleted his biceps. She was later brought in DOA, dead on arrival, with both barrels of a shotgun unloaded in her chest.

This unhappy customer continued his rampage. He found the prostitute's pimp and unloaded a few more shells from his shotgun in his direction. The pimp was well prepared. He had easily avoided the drunken man's shotgun blasts and returned six rounds, one striking him in the left chest, and the other in the neck.

He survived three surgeries, 15 pints of blood, and another attempt by the pimp on his life.

These incidents were all in one evening. Rape, sexual abuse, venereal diseases, abortion, adultery leading to murder, all were present in full and living color. I quickly came to grips with all the issues of sexual promiscuity and their devastating and cruel results. The issues of sexuality present a host of complex, divisive and dangerous situations to those in leadership positions, in our communities, in our churches, and in our families. These include the violent and grotesque forms of criminal sexuality as just mentioned, the rapidly spreading epidemic of AIDS, the teen pregancy and abortions problems, venereal diseases, adultery and divorce, addiction to pornography, homosexuality, and others.

The AIDS epidemic is a direct result of sexual immorality on the African and American continents and is potentially the worst disease problem ever to infect this planet. It has disseminated more rapidly than any sexually spread disease known to man and because we have no cure for viral infections, it has continued on its unrelenting killing spree. Estimated numbers of deaths from the AIDS virus will reach to 100 million by the end of this century. It is truly a modern-day plague of historic proportions.

The teen pregnancy problem affects one-out-of-four teen women in the United States in spite of sex education in our public school systems and the free supply of contraceptives through agencies such as Planned Parenthood. These immature young mothers are often coerced and counseled to abort the unborn child, justifying their heinous actions by claiming the mother's right to privacy. The destruction of human life through abortion has become a tragic, yet popular method of terminating many "unplanned" pregnancies.

Venereal diseases, those infections spread by sexual contact, have been known for centuries. The disease syphilis, a slow and deadly infection, killed king and pauper alike before an antibiotic cure was developed in the 1940s. In the past 30 years, a continual proliferation in the numbers and types of sexually transmitted diseases has occurred. Gonorrhea, syphilis, chlamydia, chancroid, herpes, and now AIDS, all are causing pain, destruction, and death. Even in the face of AIDS, some cities are still reporting huge increases in the numbers of cases of venereal infections.

The holy estate of marriage is regarded as the lowly penny, an object unworthy of any saving effort. Sexually based marriages last only as long as the thrill of "good sex" keeps them together. Sexual relationships may occur outside of marriage to fulfill hungering, passionate desires. This infidelity destroys the love, trust, and respect between supposedly trustworthy partners. Modern marriage vows often reflect this change in perspective, promising faithfulness until "love dies" instead of till "death do us part."

The problem of adultery and sexual relationships prior to marriage encourages "sexual abuse" and unquenchable sexual appetites. The need for sexual stimulation increases as the appetite is fed. Sexual relationships within marriage may become less and less exciting, leading to a perceived need for extra-marital "more fulfilling sex." After a while, even this sexual "escapism" doesn't quench the need for more stimulation, and the sexual addict becomes more and more addicted. Rape, incest, sexual perversions, and pornography all stem from an unquenchable sexual appetite fed by bizarre forms of sexual gratification.

The list goes on.

But possibly the most important issue generating and expanding all of the above is the issue of tolerance of sexual promiscuity within all sectors of our society. It is easy to tolerate a behavior when there is no personal damage or pain. But we must continue to remember that people are hurt, destroyed, emotionally crushed, and physically diseased by this "supposedly benign" new sexuality. It happens every day to people like you and me, and it happens because we have tolerated these sexual behaviors in our society and in our churches.

TOLERANCE AND COMPROMISE

I was on my way into the hospital lobby when I was stopped by a friend in our church.

"Hey, brother. I was really disappointed to see you compromise yourself," he pronounced in a mildly angry tone.

"I'm sorry, but I'm not sure that I understand," I said. .

"I saw you drinking one of those "Big Gulp" drinks from that pornograpy store. We're boycotting them, 'til they get rid of all that garbage. I just can't believe you would compromise yourself like that." My friend stated his points with authority.

"Thank you for your concern," I said, "but I think you missed what the pastor announced from the pulpit. He said that all those 'pornography stores' in our state have not carried those magazines for years. Drinking a 'Big Gulp' gives me a chance to thank them for not carrying that sleaze on their shelves."

We all have our ideas about compromise. Some won't compromise on legalistic matters, hair length, dress length, or sermon length. Others, such as myself, find it difficult to compromise on ideals, such as proper nutrition, excercise, and bodily care. It is important for those in the church to learn to tolerate each other and their own ideas of living and serving. But the church cannot, must not tolerate sin, or we will become disobedient servants.

The non-Christian population of the United States does not understand its level of tolerance to illicit sexual behavior. Nor does it understand the social and personal consequences of this accommodation to sin. The consequences of this tolerance have lead to the compromising of moral values in all segments of our culture.

Societal values and standards are an important determinate of our relationships. A decline in business standards has resulted in misleading advertising, need for extensive contracts, hostile take-over attempts, and insider trading scandals. A slide in judicial standards, where law is interpreted instead of upheld, has created the "malpractice lottery," suit-happy citizens, and courts that create dangerous laws and destroy basic human rights. The degeneration of sexual standards has manufactured millions of new victims through teen-pregnancy, abortion, and criminal sexuality.

For many decades, the church remained the guardian of these social standards, attaining a governing position in the hearts and minds of its citizens. But now, the traditional role of religious thought no longer reigns. We've replaced it with the secular ideologies that promote man's individual freedoms over responsible action. Pleasure-seekers who call the Judeo-Christian ethic a meaningless philosphy and a restrictor of personal freedom are really denouncing the church's ideology.

The church's position has suffered from external attacks and at the same time from division and compromise within its own ranks. Sexual standards within the church have continued to weaken as lay persons and church leaders have been seduced to accept a higher and higher level of

Plague in Our Midst

open sexual promiscuity. Even prominent leaders within the church have succumbed to sexual passions, failing the biblical test of leadership.

What church has responded to this call for "more sexuality" by denouncing it from its pulpit? Bewildered saints now call upon stunned church leaders who never received formal training in sexual attitudes and function in their seminary or undergraduate course work. Believers remain shocked at the "sinfulness and degradation" of the world. A concerted response from those in authority has been slow and limited to a few well-known voices within the media, those who call for biblical repentance from sexual sin.

The church is like the proverbial ostrich with its head buried in the sand. While the sin is hidden from view, the tail end is left exposed to be affected by the world.

Non-Christian tolerance for "changes in lifestyles" and the church's slow and apathetic response encourages "godly living" and to call sin sin has resulted in a generation of confused, misled, misinformed, and troubled young people. Many of them live in our homes, attend our Christian day-schools and belong to our churches. The life and health of our families depend upon the reponse we make to the world's call for tolerance to sexual promiscuity.

Again, reality strikes home.

CHANGING OUR COURSE

For me, it took the reality of a dear Christian friend dying from AIDS. It took the realization that sexual promiscuity was a serious problem within our churches. It took the helpless feeling that my own children and my wife were at risk. It took a great deal to realize that our course had to be changed, that we must take an active role in the solution, not the problem.

On top of the darkest, most ominous clouds, there are radiant billows gorgeously illuminated by the sun. Those clouds, representing moral perversion and rampant sexuality, can be illuminated by God's Son, who can use this dire moral situation to bring glory, possibly even revival, to this nation. What the church has been unwilling to do through preaching from the pulpit, God is able to do by the devastation of disease. We need to change our course toward a scriptural understanding of marriage and sexuality, steering toward Christ, our Direction and Destination.

Jesus Christ and His Word are the answer for these social issues, as well as for our eternal spiritual need. Though this sounds too simplistic and dogmatic for many, they cannot deny that salvation in Christ and proper grounding in the biblical principles of sexuality have changed lives.

If we are to change our course, we must gain knowledge, understanding, and wisdom concerning the biblical principles for sexual attitudes, values, functions, and marital relationships. We must indelibly etch these important principles in our thought patterns so that the Holy Spirit can use them to protect us from the world's subtle, seductive attitudes toward sexual immorality.

Most parents do not know the essential information concerning sexual function and physiology. Without this background, they find discussions related to sexuality, sexually transmitted diseases, and AIDS impossible. Yet, once they understand this information, they will find teaching their children about sexuality and dealing with sexual problems inside and outside of the family will become more manageable.

As a father whose children often copy his behavior, I have learned I am the most effective teaching tool they have when I consistently model the principles I seek to teach. If we desire to snatch our children away from the temptation of sexual promiscuity, our behavior needs to demonstrate these same biblical principles. Those in the world will be confused if we do not act upon our values, and even our own children will be unimpressed by our convictions without action.

TRAINING OUR CHILDREN

What do we tell our children when it comes to teaching them about sexual attitudes? Are we not exhorted by Scripture to train up a child in the way that he should go, and he will not depart from it? (Proverbs 22:6) What is our responsibility?

As stated before, surveys of both Christian and non-Christian young people suggest that parents are the primary source of sex education in only 20 percent of the homes. Christian homes were the same as non-Christian homes, both about 20 percent. The scriptural principle is clear that we are to train our children. But only 20 percent of Christian young people have parents who are training them in the proper values, principles and attitudes concerning heterosexual relationships and marriage. The other 80 percent are left to their own lust and devices, being trained by boyfriends, girlfriends, brothers, sisters, television, advertisements, and magazines. Some are trained by public school teachers who are not willing to make value judgments about proper and immoral sexual relationships.

Our present predicament remains. Sexual standards are declining. The church's moral leadership is questioned from within and without. Society is disobedient to God's principles and the results are being realized. Many parents know virtually nothing about human sexuality and are impotent in positively affecting our society and our children.

One simple fact should motivate us to become informed about AIDS and about sexual promiscuity within our communities and churches. The fact that should drive us to immediate action is that AIDS kills people. People — like Jay and Jenny, pastors, drug addicts, hemophiliacs, parents, children, and even grandparents; people we know, their sons or daughters, our neighbors and friends, possibly even our own family members — may die of AIDS.

This plague is not just in the slums of Harlem, the shooting galleries of Chicago, the prostitutes of Miami. It has infected those within the church by blood transfusion, by needle stick, and by promiscuous sex. If you saw 200 people today, there is a good chance that one of them has AIDS. Maybe the one you talked with, the one you rubbed shoulders with, the helpful young lady at the market, the young man who asked to rake your leaves.

It is my fervent desire that our hearts will be awakened to the gravity of this situation, as well as awakened to the dire spiritual needs that are arising. We have a great message of hope to take to those who will be afflicted, who will be humbled on their sick bed.

As well, protection for our families must also become our high priority as we teach and model biblical principles and build proper sexual attitudes into their lives. Only by our obedience to these principles of sexuality can we be assured of protection from disease and the blessing of God on our lives.

My life has been drastically changed by the plague in our midst. The way I practice medicine, the types of medical procedures that I would do in Africa, the way I handle patients, and the way I teach my children, all have or will be changed because of AIDS. My heart has been broken by the spiritual needs of thousands of people who are infected with this deadly virus and thousands more who will be. The plague of AIDS has changed my life.

Let God use the reality of this situation to change your life as well.

CHAPTER TWO
THE PLAGUE OF AIDS

My interest in AIDS led me to attend a National Conference on HIV (Human Immunodeficiency Virus), the new term for the AIDS virus. The plight of my friend Jay and some of the other patients that I have ministered to, instilled in me an intense desire to understand this disease. I needed as many tools as possible if I was to help my patients.

Many experts in AIDS research attended and were able to share some of the latest technical information about the disease, its cause, and its spread. The meeting was conducted with the usual unemotional information that is so common for medical professionals. Yet, the facts, the new information, the statistics, the truths, made many of these unemotional physicians cringe. Though we are gaining greatly in our scientific understanding, we are still a very long way from a vaccine or a treatment to cure the disease.

We all sat there numb as the facts penetrated our hopes,

as we understood the danger to our families, our patients and our country.

The power of this epidemic has even changed the minds of our leaders. The speakers, government officials, scientists, physicians and those working to understand this epidemic almost unanimously stated that the only way to stop this disease is to abstain from sexual promiscuity and from IV drugs. I was amazed to see these amoral scientists make such a major ideological shift. This is a monumental move in the right direction for these experts and a move they know in their heart is right.

The most important task of this book is to give you the cold, hard facts about AIDS, about sexuality and about how we can teach and protect our families from this disease. Here is some of the most recent information, given in plain, simple language so that each of us will begin to understand this plague in our midst.

THE DEVASTATION OF AIDS

We are facing today the most deadly disease ever known to mankind! No other pestilence, war, environmental factor short of nuclear holocaust has the potential of killing 100 million persons by the end of this century.

The AIDS infection is presently epidemic in the United States, in Haiti, and in many countries of Africa, quickly spreading through promiscuous sexual contacts and through use of illegal intravenous drugs. The current estimate of individuals infected in the United States, given by a number of health authorities, suggests that 1.5-million Americans are presently infected with the virus; 87,000 have already tested positively for the disease; 60,000 have clinical cases of HIV infection. Ten million persons worldwide are presently infected with the virus with future estimates as high as 100 million by the year 1993.

Though the numbers are staggering to the imagination, AIDS is still a disease of individual victims. Each has had his

Plague in Our Midst

life sapped prematurely, his family devastated, his hope destroyed. Children of drug-using parents are born with the virus and develop painful infections at early ages. Wives die because of a husband's infidelity. Hemophiliacs and surgical patients who must rely upon a tainted blood supply contract the disease through life-saving treatments. Innocent travelers who unknowingly received an injection from a "reused" needle have contracted AIDS while abroad. Adolescents who are tempted and who succumb to the pleasures of sex or the highs of drug usage have become infected from one such episode of sin.

AIDS is not just a disease of hard-core junkies in the "shooting galleries" of New York, prostitutes in the streets of Chicago, promiscuous homosexuals in the bath houses of San Fransisco. It is a disease that can and will affect all Americans if the epidemic is not stopped.

BASIC INFORMATION ABOUT AIDS

The term AIDS is an acronym, a word formed from the first letters of its meaning. AIDS stands for Acquired Immune Deficiency Syndrome. Acquired means that the disease is passed from person to person. The immune system is the body's defense system, made up of blood cells, skin, liver, spleen, lymph nodes and other organs. It fights to rid the body of invading pests and to heal the body when it's damaged. In AIDS, a deficiency occurs. The body's immune system becomes ineffective and unable to protect itself from normal illnesses.

The syndrome of AIDS is caused by a virus, the HIV virus or Human Immunodeficiency Virus. This virus and other similar viruses have been discovered in persons in the United States and in many other countries in the world, especially in Africa. The presence of the virus is detected when blood samples from the infected individual show antibodies for HIV.

The HIV or AIDS virus is passed through three main

routes: sexual contact with an infected person, sharing intravenous needles with an infected person, and receiving an infected blood transfusion.

Intimate sexual contact, homosexual or heterosexual, can spread the virus from the infected person to an uninfected person. Homosexual relations, either rectal or oral intercourse, spread the virus, allowing easy entry through the mucous membranes, or through tears in the rectum. Common sexual practices within the homosexual community, such as having sex with multiple partners, ignoring disease protection devices, and sexual intercourse that tears tissue, have rapidly spread the virus from person to person.

Intravenous drug users have also become infected, passing the virus with shared needles. Homosexual and prostitute drug abusers originally passed the virus to other non-homosexual drug users and now the virus is rampant within that community. Those who are addicted to IV drugs have their own social-support system built upon sharing drugs, needles, joints and sex. Unfortunately they share their diseases as well, such as Hepatitis B. Clean needles will make little difference because drug users thrive on social cameraderie, supporting one another through shared needles or through sexual relations.

A number of hemophiliacs have contracted AIDS through blood transfusions because they need blood and clotting products to correct a deficiency in their own clotting mechanism. Homosexual drug abusers and prostitutes in larger cities sell their blood to pay for a fix. Presently, all persons are screened before giving their blood. As well, blood banks have started extensive campaigns to test all blood given to patients. Yet recent studies show that the infection can be present for as long as 12 months before antibody tests become positive. This creates uncertainty as to the safety of transfused blood. Clotting factors are now heat-treated to decrease the risk of spread to hemophiliacs.

RISK FACTORS

The term "risk factor" is used to suggest what a person is or is not doing that makes him susceptible to a disease. Homosexual feelings are not a risk, whereas sex with multiple homosexual partners is. Abusing oral tranquilizers is not a risk, but injecting drugs with a shared needle is. Having a sexual affair is a risk factor especially when no disease protection is used.

The AIDS virus is found in high concentrations in semen, in vaginal mucous secretions, and in the blood. The virus can thus be passed from person to person when these fluids are passed during sexual intercourse or with transfusions. AIDS can also be passed from an infected mother to an unborn child through the placental nutrition system and through breast milk as well.

AIDS INFECTION

The AIDS virus is both a direct cause of disease and a factor that allows other deadly diseases to invade, attack, and destroy a human individual. The HIV invades the immune system and often remains dormant for months to years after the initial sexual contact. It appears to hide within the T-lymphocytes where it cannot be attacked and destroyed. It hides and attacks other tissues as well, such as the brain. The virus unwraps its protein coat once it is inside the cell. It joins its genetic instructions with the genetic instructions of the cell. Every time a new cell is produced, new viral particles are produced as well. The body's defense system would have to attack and destroy itself, or self-destruct, to rid itself of the AIDS virus.

AIDS does much of its damage by destroying the body's immune or defense function. This allows other disease processes, such as serious infections of the lung or cancers like Kaposi's sarcoma, to invade the body and destroy it. Without an immune system, simple infections can be deadly. AIDS victims have died from bacterial, viral, and protazoal infections of the lungs and of the brain, infections disseminated through the body and from various cancers.

The virus becomes active in most of the people who have been infected, possibly all. Of those who caught the virus through homosexual contact, 25-50 percent will get an active case of the disease within five years, rapidly dying from the opportunistic infections or from cancer. The sad fact remains, however, that all present projections of the disease suggest that 100 percent will eventually die from immune compromise. There is always some hope that all will not die from the disease, but there are no guarantees.

SIGNS AND SYMTOMS

After the initial sexual contact, the infected person notices no signs or symptoms for months to years. That is why AIDS is so dangerous and so easily spread. Most people who have the virus have no symptoms and continue to pass the disease through sexual relations or through intravenous drug usage long before they get sick.

Those individuals who have the antibody present in their blood have been infected with the AIDS virus and are contagious to other persons by sexual or blood spread.

The media has used the term "exposed" to make the public believe these individuals will never get an active case of AIDS, leading to destruction of their immune function. The more proper definition would be "infected" as all these people are contagious and spread death through promiscuous behavior.

Two forms of active disease are described, AIDS and ARC (AIDS related complex). In the ARC form, the person tests positively for the AIDS virus, but has a less severe form of the disease with symptoms of fever, weight-loss, night sweats, skin rashes, diarrhea, tiredness, lack of resistance to infections, and swollen lymph nodes. Full-blown AIDS infections are diagnosed by the presence of certain types of opportunistic infections or tumors, or serious cases of more common infections such as shingles, TB, CMV, or mononucleosis.

Besides the devastating infections that occur, some symptoms come from the active destruction of tissues by the AIDS virus. Damage to the nervous system shows itself in memory loss, indifference, loss of coordination, partial paralysis, or mental disorders. These symptoms are similar to other "slow viruses" that have been discovered, and they are similar to other degenerative mental conditions such as Alzheimer's disease.

THE FUTURE OF AIDS

On paper, AIDS easily has the potential of becoming the world's worst disease plague to date. Some have estimated that worldwide, if the AIDS virus continues to spread at its presently increasing rate, more than 100 million people could be infected with the virus and die from its complications. More than 60,000 persons in the United States are presently known to have AIDS or to have died from complications related to AIDS. More than 1.5 million Americans are infected with the virus now and worldwide figures reach 10 million people. If the disease continues on its present exponential rate of increase, 100 million people with AIDS may be a very conservative estimate.

The situation on the African continent is frightful. Some of the countries in eastern Africa have rates of infection from five percent to 20 percent. Promiscuous sexuality on that continent has spread the disease to both males and females. Some tribes are more severely stricken than others, as promiscuity remains within the tribe. In the cities, however, sexual promiscuity is even worse. One study showed 90 percent of all prostitutes in one area were infected, as were 30 percent of their partners.

The AIDS spread within many of these third world cultures is almost guaranteed to run wild with so little media education and so much promiscuous sexuality. The money to accomplish testing, reporting and contact tracing is virtually non-existent. What is left to stop the epidemic in Africa?

Other countries, such as Haiti, have high rates of infection as well. One group of Haitian immigrants to the U.S. was tested and shown to have an infection rate of 40 percent. Most of the general estimates for Haiti and other infected countries suggest a much lower infection rate than this.

The potential spread of AIDS infections within these "hot beds" of eastern Africa, Haiti, the United States, and others depends upon the decrease in promiscuous sexual behavior, the education of the masses about AIDS and, most importantly, the testing of appropriate individuals and blood products. The staggering potential of 100 million persons dead from the AIDS virus by the year 2000 should stir us to action.

PREVENTION OF AIDS

To understand the possibilities of contagious disease prevention, we must first define levels of contact. "Intimate" contact is defined as sexual contact and the sharing or transfering of bodily fluids. "Close" contact is defined as living with an individual, caring or cleaning bodily fluids or wastes, eating with and/or sleeping in the same bed with the individual on multiple occasions. "Casual" contact is touching a person's body or touching an object that has touched the person a single time.

Hepatitis B is a viral disease that is spread by intimate contact, sexual secretions, transfusions, and rarely by saliva or close contact with an infected person. The vectors of spread appear to be identical between the AIDS virus and Hepatitis B. As it has been proven that close contact with the Hepatitis B virus can spread the infection, it would be wise to take precautions to avoid close contact with persons with the AIDS virus as well. This has been shown to be necessary with a small number of probable cases of close contact spread of the AIDS virus. This may be the reason why seven percent of all AIDS victims do not know where they contracted their infection.

It is impossible to prove casual contact as a source of disease spread. But casual contact may become a means of spread when the virus mutates and becomes more stable outside of the body. Casual spread becomes likely when many more persons become infected with and shed the virus in the environment.

Prevention of the spread of AIDS is assured through sexual abstinence and by abstinence from IV drug usage. Close contacts of persons with AIDS should take the same precautions that health care workers use when dealing with patients with Hepatitis B — protection from bodily fluids and blood transfers. Close contacts must also take precautions not to contract cases of other diseases carried by the AIDS victim — anything from colds to pneumonia.

POLITICS AND AIDS

Never has the conquest of an epidemic contagious disease been so completely stifled and complicated by the strength of a minority political movement. The homosexual lobby has opportunistically used the disease of AIDS to further its claim for social legitimacy by changing the definition of discrimination. The blatant promotion of its anti-social values through this disease makes no common sense, but it has struck at the heart-strings of many liberal officials who wish to help this group for personal gain.

Claiming discrimination on the basis of AIDS for all homosexuals is like claiming discrimination against all smokers because they are likely to be afflicted with pneumonia. Are drug addicts discriminated against because they contract Hepatitis B through illegal use of narcotics? Is it right for prostitutes to claim discrimination because they will contract venereal disease? Should school children strike and picket in Washington, D.C. because they are likely to contract strep throat? This line of reasoning remains absolutely absurd.

The special interest groups that are promoting these disciminatory claims have effectively stopped the institution of the public health statutes from stemming the tide of the AIDS epidemic. The political strength of the "gay left" has stopped almost all state legislation that would call for the testing of risk groups, the reporting of positive tests to public health authorities, and the tracing of all known contacts, all proven effective in halting the spread of disease. Only a few states have been able to overcome "gay-rights" pressure by passing such laws. California, a gay stronghold, has passed laws which prohibit the reporting of a positive AIDS test even to a family member or another health care professional, the very people who need to know for their own safety.

Epidemics can only be brought under control when reasonable means of precaution are taken to prevent their spread. We have no cure for the AIDS virus. We have no vaccine to prevent its spread. We have no effective treatments to stop the disease once an individual is infected. The only means left to bring this disease under control are the public health laws that utilize confidential testing, case reporting, and contact identification to stop diseases from spreading.

EDUCATION ABOUT AIDS

Some people believe that education is the cornerstone in the attack against the AIDS epidemic. This erroneous belief supposes that people, especially young adults, will voluntarily change their sexual behaviors when presented with the facts and responsibilities. The sad truth is that certain types of addictive behaviors, such as sex or drug use, are extremely difficult to change even when people have a desire to change. Other difficulties arise when some of us tell young people to abstain from promiscuity, while others of us promote free sex without protection on all television programming. Most young people will follow the path of least resistance and do "what comes naturally."

Education has proved ineffective in other health areas where fatal consequences result, such as smoking and intravenous drug usage. We have waged a massive educational offensive on the issue of drunken driving, and the results have been somewhat positive. But they are far less than optimal. Obviously, printed educational material will be worthless for the illiterate, the blind and other groups. The deaf will probably not be catered to in any educational campaign. Even experts in media education realize that education alone is ineffective in halting the AIDS epidemic.

The only way this society will slow the spread of AIDS to millions of other innocent victims will be through the enactment of proper public health laws, testing, reporting, and contact tracing; through a massive public education effort stressing abstinence from sex and IV drug usage; and through the compassionate response by the church, those who will meet the needs of these dying persons.

NEED FOR COMPASSION

This information may not be that alarming to many who read this book. It wasn't as devastating to me until I knew someone who had the disease. The information about AIDS may not become a reality to you as well, until you personally know a victim.

Let me share with you some of the people that I have taken care of — people who are dying or who are now dead of AIDS. Their faces may be very familiar.

This had been the third hospital admission for Carol in the last three months. She had diarrhea that would not stop, and her cough had gotten worse. As I sat at her bedside, she shared with me how she had contracted AIDS.

At the age of 18, she had just finished high school and

was starting to work at a local department store. Though she had one other episode of "sex," she had never had intercourse. She was wanting to save herself for "Mr. Right."

One afternoon late, just before closing time, Robert made his appearance. Within two to three weeks they were talking about marriage and sleeping together on a regular basis. Their relationship seemed to be growing until a fight over moving to a different, nearby town caused Robert to move out. Carol was initially devastated, but she quickly forgot about him.

She remained single, did not marry, and did not have sex with any other boyfriends. Three years later she was dying of AIDS.

As I sat talking with this patient, her eyes sunken from the dehydration, her skin gray and her voice weak, she asked over and over again what her chances were. She understood that her sexual affair led to this disease, and she had personally sought God's forgiveness. What she could not comprehend was the fact that medicine could not cure AIDS, only some of the infections.

"We know about computers and space travel, how come we can't cure AIDS?"

Even though she had the best of medical care, including some experimental drugs for AIDS, she died of Pneumocystis carinii pneumonia about six months later. I have never felt more helpless, more inadequate as a physician than during my talks with Carol.

Terry was a young drug addict I first met in the emergency room. He had used heroin for four years and was unwilling to seek help for his addiction. During the last two years he had spent eight months in New York City, staying with some friends.

I had to admit him to the hospital for fevers of 104 degrees, large, swollen, painful lymph nodes everywhere, and a rash — a "shingles" rash — all over his body. He was in excruciating pain.

Plague in Our Midst

We put him on the strongest antibiotics we had, and his fever did start to come down; but the excruciating pain continued. He was given injection after injection of the best narcotic pain medications, all without relief. He finally walked out of the hospital so he could treat himself with heroin.

Terry's AIDS test was positive, but the test did not come back from the laboratory until he was on the streets. We attempted to find him, to tell him, but were unable. What got to me was not just Terry and his discomfort. It was his girlfriend. She had never taken any IV drugs and was hoping to save Terry from his "wicked" addiction. Now she would be the loser with a 50 percent chance of contracting and dying from AIDS. I can still remember the blind love in her eyes for Terry.

Ray was a 56-year-old lawyer, married with two grown children. His law practice was thriving, and his marriage had never been better. He was planning on taking early retirement with his wife, but that never happened. In 1983 he had severe abdominal pain and was rushed to the hospital for gall bladder surgery. Blood was lost during the procedure and two units were given.

The summer of 1987, one week after Ray's 56th birthday, he became ill with swollen lymph nodes and pneumonia. Over the next three months he lost weight rapidly and was hospitalized five times for infections. He became confused and very weak. The last days of his life were spent in a hospital, babbling, with a fever of 105 degrees, unable to recognize his family, very short of breath.

I still don't know if Ray was saved.

There are others. Look closely at the faces of these victims. The two-year-old child, screaming from the pain of shingles, all over his little body; the wife who must deal with the emotional pain of an unfaithful husband along with the pain and infections from AIDS; the thin, pale, emaciated face of an AIDS victim, looking like a survivor from a Nazi "death" camp. The emotional pain of these victims who are assured of months to years of suffering without knowing the hour it will end.

Though the major spread of this epidemic has occurred through homosexual lust and addiction to pleasure, there must be an outpouring of forgiving compassion if we will be allowed the privilege of sharing Christ with these addicts of self-indulgence. Did not Christ himself reach out to the very dregs of Roman-Judeo society, the sick, the infirmed, the poor, the forgotten. His compassion was evident in His preaching against sin and in His love for the sinner through word and action.

It didn't take many of these faces — precious lives wasted in sinful practices — to touch my heart. It probably won't take many to break yours as well. We need to share the compassion of Christ with as many as God allows to cross our paths.

Our compassionate response for the AIDS victim can move us to appropriate and caring action. First, we must firmly speak out against sin and against the sinful ideals and philosophies that are enslaving millions of people. Second, we must lovingly reach out to all the victims of AIDS by offering them the hope of salvation through Jesus Christ. Third, we must teach our children what Scripture has to say about sexuality, about marriage, about obedience, and about the blessings and protection that comes when we follow God's direction for our lives.

CHAPTER THREE
THE BIBLICAL PERSPECTIVE OF SEXUALITY

God has ordained one relationship on this earth to be more special, blessed, holy, exalted than all other interpersonal relationships — that of the marriage bond. To God, marriage was so important that He uses Christ's bond to the church to portray this relationship:

"Husbands, love your wives, just as Christ loved the church and gave himself up for her to make her holy, cleansing her by the washing with water through the word, and to present her to himself as a radiant church, without stain or wrinkle or any other blemish, but holy and blameless." Ephesians 5:25-27 (NIV)

The marriage relationship, as many authors, lecturers and pastors have stated, is the foundation used by God to build relationships with Himself. He uses this foundation to demonstrate many principles about husband-wife relations, parent-child relations, and Christian-sinner relations. Marriage teaches a scriptural pattern of behavior that can be applied to all human inter-relationships, especially the sexual relationship.

Paul and Alisa were told by their secular friends that their marriage was "one-in-a-million." They had been married for 10 years and were blessed with three children.

The family was Paul's first priority. He had accepted a 40-percent pay cut so that he could have time off to spend with his wife and children. Alisa was a full-time mother, caring for the three children and supporting Paul's work schedule and business. She was always busily making a craft for a friend, a cake for the fellowship night or helping drive a friend or senior saint to the store.

Christie, their four-year-old, likes to brag about her parents.

"Mom and dad sure love each other. They never fight. They always help each other. They never complain, and they pray about everything."

Paul and Alisa decided early in their marriage to put their marriage partner first in their prayer life, their thoughts, and their desires. Their relationship and how they treat their children is based on role models offered by scripture.

I have the privilege of knowing this young couple personally, as both friends and patients. Though their marriage is a great gift of God, built upon His principles, I have also seen the great amount of prayer, diligence and discipline it takes for Paul and Alisa to live in such harmony.

Let's look at some scriptural definitions of sexual behavior through studying the biblical roles for the husband and wife.

THE HUSBAND'S ROLE

Within the marriage relationship, God has ordained a head, the husband, within the family.

Plague in Our Midst

> *"Wives, submit to your husbands as to the Lord. For the husband is the head of the wife as Christ is the head of the church, his body, of which he is the Savior." Ephesians 5:22-23 (NIV)*

The stability of the family depends upon the husband and his proper relationship as head of the family. The constant battling between husband and wife over issues of control, who decides on the finances, who regulates the children's behavior and who is responsible for initiating communications, will produce emotional and spiritual strife in both parents and children. Everything rises or falls, grows or dwindles on the husband's leadership.

Imagining the difficulties of an unstable family should teach us some lessons concerning the stability of our personal relationship with our heavenly Father. If we are constantly bickering over control of our lives instead of allowing God to lead, guide and direct us through the Holy Spirit, we too will reap the results of our folly. A strong, trusting, loving, nurturing relationship is built between God and ourselves if we allow Him to control. Unlike a contentious spouse, God is too loving to "fight" for control of lives entrusted to His care, but He carefully and lovingly allows us to make our own mistakes until we realize our need for His leadership.

Leadership of the husband in the family and leadership of God the Father in our lives is essential for spiritual maturity and growth. Leadership has a price. Husbands are called to love their wives as Christ loved the church and gave himself for its redemption. Christ gave His very life for His bride. Husbands too are called to give all — their possessions, their time, their talents, their love, even sacrificing self if necessary for the wife. They are called to obediently follow Christ, instilling faith in all aspects of family life.

Do we see many Christ-centered homes today that are fulfilling this lofty goal for the family? How many husbands will sacrifice a career for the love of their spouses? How many men would sacrifice the "Superbowl" for a quiet afternoon with their mates or families? How many fathers would stay home to take care of the children when their wives are too ill to manage?

Men as husbands are called to give everthing within their power to support, love, nurture, care, and cultivate their marital relationship and their children. This self-sacrifical attitude toward the mates, that is patterned after Christ's self-sacrifical death for the church, will cause God's blessings to fill the home. Self-sacrifice demonstrates to the wife and children the ultimate example of Christ's love that will blossom into a loving, God-centered, Spirit-filled home. This is the supreme example for which Christian husbands must strive.

THE WIFE'S ROLE

The wife is called to be submissive to the husband, just as the husband is submissive to Christ. Leadership is not in question; for, by submission to the head of the household, the wife is showing her love and respect for her husband and her heavenly Father. A spiritually sensitive husband will allow the wife to control those areas of the home where she is best suited to govern, while the husband remains responsible for all that occurs within the home before God.

The husband shows his love for the family by leading and taking responsibility for all activities with sensitivity, sacrificing his needs for the welfare of his family. The wife faithfully shows her love for her family by supporting the household program of the husband, diligently caring for every detail and sensitively meeting the emotional and spiritual needs of the family. The wife sacrifices self in obedience to God's plan for the family.

This relationship, between Christ and the Church and between husband and wife, embodies the essential principles for Christian sexual attitudes, obedience, self-sacrifice and faith.

CHRISTIAN SEXUAL ATTITUDES

What are sexual attitudes and how are Christian sexual attitudes different from secular, worldly sexual attitudes?

Sexual attitudes are an individual's understanding of male and female relationships. We see and become comfortable with certain types of relationships and certain qualities within the relationship. We become uncomfortable when we see unfamiliar or strange characteristics.

Parents are the first male-female relationship that we come to know. We observed how our parents behaved toward each other — their communication, their affection, their habits, their hobbies, their emotions, and their love. Later, we observed other men and women and how they acted toward each other. Through these observations we began to formulate our own opinions, based on the sum of our experiences and seasoned with the values and principles that we observed in parents.

An individual's sexual attitude is the summation of all experiences and observations, tempered with family values and principles. Worldly values creep into our sexual attitudes through observations of excessively affectionate or sexually oriented relationships. We may observe these relationships in person or vicariously through the media such as magazines, advertisements, movies, music lyrics, books, television, videos, etc. These worldly attitudes promote sex for pleasure, enticing the viewer "to believe" in self-indulgence.

Christian sexual attitudes are based on our understanding of Scripture and not in the world's seductive self-gratification through recreational sexuality. Born-again children of God live by a new set of rules that dictate our wants and desires. Discipline and self-control become important qualities for maintaining proper prayer and study habits. As the word saturates every corner of our being, our fleshly attitudes come under scrutiny and we let them be refined into new, Spirit-filled principles. The Word restructures our sexual attitudes and elevates Christian principles above the worldly ones we've previously learned.

"You were taught, with regard to your former way of life, to put off your old self, which is being corrupted by its deceitful desires; to be made new in the attitude of your minds; and to put on the new self, created to be like God in true righteousness and holiness." Ephesians 4:22-24 (NIV)

What joy we will receive when our old ideas of sexuality are recreated to conform with the mind of Christ.

THE MARITAL SEXUAL RELATIONSHIP

The Christian view of sexuality is far more than the act of procreation itself. In fact, within a marriage relationship, sexual relations make up only a small fraction of the time spent together. Scripture supports the importance and function of the sexual consummation within a Christian union.

The marital sexual relationship nurtures the formation of "the one flesh" as the couple follows the scriptural ideals of leadership and submission. Each member of this blessed union invests trust and submission in the other member, knitting together a relationship where one cannot hurt without pain in the other, or rejoices without joy in the other. Spiritually, there becomes no sweeter fellowship, no greater encourager, no deeper faith than that found in the other.

Sex within marriage melts two separate individuals into a relationship that acts as one. Christ's death on the cross virtually does the same for the church, as His death redeems the church, bringing it into oneness with the Father.

"'For this reason (marriage) a man shall leave his father and mother and be united to his wife, and the two will become one flesh. This is a profound mystery — but I am talking about Christ and the church." Ephesians 5:31-32 Genesis 2:24 (NIV)

In His boundless wisdom, the Father created a situation within marriage that molds two souls into one, gives intense pleasure and builds trust and growth into the relationship. These are again, similar virtues of our spiritual relationship with the Father through Christ. Our striving should be for oneness with our Lord, through prayer and study, through a deeper trust in Him, and through following His direction. The growth in our relationship with the Father gives us a pleasurable peace that passes all understanding.

The understanding we obtain from studying the New Testament concerning sexual attitudes is that sex is ordained for the marriage and within the marriage as it is intended to blend two persons into oneness. Sex is not the marriage, but only the cement that holds the bricks of communication, trust, self-sacrifice, leadership, submission, respect and love together.

Sex within the marriage builds the relationship. Sex outside the confines of marriage defies the principles that govern this special relationship.

CONSEQUENCES OF EXTRA-MARITAL SEX

Contrasting sexual relationships within marriage and extra-marital relationships will help us visualize the self-destructive characteristics of self-gratification and the blessings of following God's perfect laws.

As previously stated, sexual intercourse within marriage allows the individual to sacrifice all for the spouse, to give that which is most intimate for the reason of building love, trust and oneness. Sexual intercourse outside of marriage is often accomplished for short-term affection, desire or lust. There is no commitment to build a relationship, but only to obtain pleasure from the act. Intercourse becomes a tool of pleasure, like a glass of beer or a joint of marijuana. As with any self-indulgent, self-stimulating act, the need or desire for illicit sex increases. Sexual relationships outside of marriage create sex-for-self instead of self-sacrifice for the spouse.

David is a Christian newlywed who has been working for a secular trucking firm for more than three years. During that time he has been exposed to pornography in the office as well as while traveling to distant cities. He initally was satisfied with milder forms of pornography, but now he seeks out "hardcore" films and magazines to fulfill that desire.

The guilt that David experienced over his desires for these grotesque and violent pictures was tremendous and it has led him to seek professional counseling. At one session, David admitted to a sexual relationship with a prostitute after using pornography.

Shortly after their marriage, David's wife found out about his habit by accident. Now she fears that when they are together, David will be thinking about a pornographic image instead of her.

David's example demonstrates the principle of "sex-for-self." The stronger the "addiction" for self-pleasure, the more the individual craves any instrument that creates a "high," such as alcohol, recreational drugs, prescription drugs, suggestive music, pornography, lustful novels, etc.

In relationships, extra-marital sex is a strongly destructive force, disintegrating the fidelity within the marriage relationship. Honesty about previous sexual exploits in a dating situation often slams the door on a future relationship. However, with the dangers of AIDS it becomes essential to be honest about previous sexual episodes before the marriage commitment is made so that testing may be accomplished, or a safer relationship begun. Premarital sexual revelations give the perception that "my spouse-to-be didn't love me enought to save himself for me."

Adulterous relationships within marriage are grounds for serious emotional distress. The faithful spouse is crushed by the lack of trust, loyalty, care, commitment from the one that was given "all that I have."

Numerous sexually transmitted diseases are brought to an unsuspecting spouse through marital infidelity. AIDS has killed both the offending and the innocent spouse who was unaware that any promiscuous relationship was occurring. Herpes, gonorrhea, chlamydia, and other infections are spreading through adultery as well.

Sex within marriage fosters marital growth; personal comfort and safety; a warm, loving, respectful home—all part of a growing relationship. Premarital sex casts doubts and fears on the marital commitments, the spouse always wondering if it could happen in marriage as well. Adultery not only destroys trust and commitment but loads the partners with emotional guilt and often ruins the marriage.

Growth versus ruin is an easy choice for those who desire God's best in their lives. Following God's principles will bring prosperity, success and growth to the individual, family or church. Acts of immorality that are accomplished against God's principles bring guilt, despair and ruin to the individual, family or church.

ATTITUDES OF THE HEART

The heart attitude, the ideals and thoughts of the person concerning relationships, remains God's perfect standard when judging individuals, and sin.

"You have heard that is was said, 'Do not commit adultery.' But I tell you that anyone who looks at a woman lustfully has already committed adultery with her in his heart." Matthew 5:27,28 (NIV)

The sin has been committed when our sexual desires are out of control and we seek available outlets for sexual frustration. Thus, sexual intercourse with an extra-marital partner is just as sinful as dwelling on the thoughts that seek such relationships.

The Old Testament speaks specifically against the sin of adultery. The seventh commandment, "You shall not commit adultery," deals with the act of extramarital sex and places it on the "Ten Most Despicable" list of human behavior. This is repeated from Exodus to Revelation, always listing adultery as a violation of God's laws and principles.

Through the prophets, adultery aquires a different, more spiritual understanding, that broadens its definition and widens its impact. God, through the prophet Jeremiah, speaks to His "chosen ones," the children of Israel:

> "...for their rebellion is great and their backslidings many. Why should I forgive you? Your children have forsaken me and sworn by gods that are not gods. I supplied all their needs, yet they committed adultery and thronged to the house of prostitutes." Jeremiah 5:6,7 (NIV)

God the Father, as a husband to the children of Israel, has been provoked to anger by His "bride" through her adulterous behavior, her worshiping idols, her intermarrying with other peoples and her forsaking the leadership that she needed. We are taught through this prophecy that personally setting aside the principles of God is as much adultery on a spiritual plane as sleeping with another is adultery on a physical plane. Guarding our relationship with God, keeping it pure and holy, is essential to preventing spiritual adultery.

Fornication, sexual relations prior to or instead of marriage, is also decried in many areas of scripture as an act against the sovereignty of God; and, as spiritual adultery, is aligned with idolatry.

> "Put to death, therefore, whatever belongs to your earthly nature: sexual immorality (fornication), impurity, lust, evil desires and greed, which is idolatry. Because of these the wrath of God is coming." Colossians 3:5,6 (NIV)

CELIBACY

Marriage is ordained by God as the premier relationship for human personal and spiritual growth. Are any alternatives given within the context of Scripture for those who cannot, will not, or are led not to marry?

The apostle Paul discusses the option of celibacy in detail:

Plague in Our Midst

> "Now to the unmarried and the widows I say: It is good for them to stay unmarried, as I am. But if they cannot control themselves, they should marry, for it is better to marry than to burn with passion." I Corinthians 7:8,9 (NIV)

> "I would like you to be free from concern. An unmarried man is concerned about the Lord's affairs — how he can please the Lord. But a married man is concerned about the affairs of this world — how he can please his wife — and his interests are divided. An unmarried woman or virgin is concerned about the Lord's affairs: Her aim is to be devoted to the Lord in both body and spirit. But a married woman is concerned about the affairs of this world — how she can please her husband. I am saying this for your own good, not to restrict you, but that you may live in a right way in undivided devotion to the Lord." I Corinthians 7:32-35 (NIV)

The heart attitude is again the important prerequisite for celibacy. If the individual is so intent upon serving the Lord, then the Lord Himself becomes the constant companion for that individual and there is no need for a physical partner. The attitude of complete spiritual sacrifice is the key.

The celibate individual does not have the physical marriage relationship from which to learn many of the truths concerning his or her spiritual relationship. However, the Holy Spirit can teach that person through Scripture, through observing other family relationships within the church and through maintaining personal relationships with parents.

Paul also makes clear that the passionate desires, if harbored without release, may cause grave injury to the cause of Christ through immoral behavior. His suggestion is to marry to prevent lust from coming to sinful fruit. He also warns against marrying foolishly, creating an unequal yoke with a mate who is not a believer (II Corinthians 6:14). Though if one becomes a believer after marriage, there is no reason for divorce as the unbelieving spouse is sanctified through the believing spouse (I Corinthians 7:12-14). There is also opportunity to win that unbelieving spouse through the exemplary behavior and love of the believing spouse (I Peter 3:1).

Biblical principles are the beginning of all wisdom, when it comes to our relationship with God, to our marital relationship and to our sexual relationship with our spouse. As a physician who desires the best for my patients, I pray that you would fill this spiritual prescription, the principles of sexuality, to protect and prevent damage from promiscuity.

The most descriptive terms I can use to describe these biblical principles for sexuality are pure and sufficient — pure because they are simple and not cluttered with comparisons of what is "normal" or abnormal sexuality; sufficient because God has given them and they are perfect guidelines for our behavior. They lose their purity and sufficiency when we add man's knowledge to these principles, when we compare sexual habits, when we strive for sexual prowess, when we seek only to please ourselves. These are the hallmarks of worldly sexuality.

One great sorrow that I have as a physician comes when a prescription is ignored and the patient suffers. All I can do amounts to nothing if the patient decides he wants to suffer. The same is true for the patient who decides to follow the world's prescription for sexuality and its principles of selfish sexual fulfillment.

CHAPTER FOUR
The World's Sexuality

The setting is a steaming bathroom, a misty bar room, a cool night on a city street. The scenery is back lit, with haze. The actors are young and extremely attractive — one male, one female.

The scenes flash quickly from clothing being thrown on a chair to the woman waiting in the bar, sipping her beer. The smiles are seductive as they "think" about meeting each other. The music is heavy rock, filled with a pulsating beat. Interspersed between the desire — man for woman, woman for man — are shots of the tantalizing product, being poured, being sipped, being admired. All of the scenes are meant to elicit sexual arousal in the mind and to link arousal to drinking a particular beer.

Images of desire for the opposite sex have changed radically within the past 30 years. The coy, shy smile of the smartly dressed lady in the 1950s elicited a very positive response among males viewing her picture. The subtlety of this approach to sexuality, however, has been lost completely. Today, the female is dressed so that parts of her anatomy are extremely alluring and visible, her smile openly seductive, her postures and movements connote desire and availability for immediate sexual relations. The arousal brought on by this approach to visual advertisements and entertainment is nothing short of pornography; yet it has become a tolerated part of watching a sporting event, a movie or viewing television.

This new openness toward sexual displays is directly responsible for the increase in promiscuous behavior and the resultant increase in venereal diseases and sexual problems. I know that this is true because of the questions that adults and teens ask about sexuality in my office. They often justify their actions to me by comparing them to TV, to adult behaviors or other friends' actions.

A young man came into my office recently with the symptoms of gonorrhea. He stated that both he and his girlfriend were Christians but had not yet talked about marriage. They had attended a movie, an explicit movie, before their sexual escapades. When I asked him whether he considered he could pick up AIDS, his reply was no. He thought he could trust her. He also thought that birth control pills protected them from AIDS. When I asked him about the reasons for being sexually active, he mentioned movies, friends, and birth control as reasons why it was acceptable to have sex before marriage.

How did society's opinion of sexuality change so completely and so rapidly, away from the Judeo-Christian ethic to absolute hedonism? What has the church's role been in allowing this slide to take place?

A SEXUAL CONCENSUS

The general concensus of our society since the signing of the Declaration of Independence to the late 1940s has been a conservative understanding of sexual relationships. Marriage was important; divorce a social stigma. Extra-marital affairs were uncommon, as was pre-marital sexual intercourse. Though these "sexually immoral" relationships were still found, their numbers were far less than at present. Religious ideologies and teachings alone controlled the reins of society's young stallions.

The slide toward liberalization of sexual attitudes took a steep turn in the 1950s along with other cultural changes such as "Rock and Roll," the scientific explosion, and the "me" generation. Sexual freedom became a rallying cry for those who were dissatisfied with governmental policies, traditional family relationships, the draft and social norms. Sexual promiscuity initially was more a symptom of openly rebellious attitudes toward the "establishment," rather than an actual movement in and of itself.

Western culture — the United States, Canada, and Europe — has become involved in this change of sexual perspective more openly than other cultures because of personal freedom and the ever-present media. The wealthy of all cultures tend to follow the materialistic lead of western culture, taking on many of the social and business customs. The elite in each culture play the games of money, sex, and power as a means of prestige.

Why has the sexual concensus of western society changed from a conservative to hedonistic view? Two reasons.

First, young people rebelled against the traditional values, institutions and structures within society during the sixties and seventies. Parental values were thrown out and with it, the prominence of Judeo-Christian principles. Second, the entertainment industry experimented with new values, ones that portray more open, suggestive sexuality. Without the restricting influences of parental values, they found it more stimulating than plots, travelogues, and classics. They found a large and eager market in these discontented young adults, a market they would learn to exploit.

The church's stature was decreasing because of this

questioning of values and sexuality was increasing the stimulation-level of entertainment. As these Judeo-Christian values were being removed from the social norm, what else besides sin would fill that void.

This new sexuality then infiltrated the advertising industry as well as the general entertainment industry. Pornography, visual and written, became more plentiful, more open and graphic. Through all of this, the church's voice was silent. Without resistance, the sexual consensus moved toward open sexuality.

THE CHURCH'S CALL

As stated in scripture, it was the purpose of the cross (and is the purpose of all believers) to call sinners away from sin to a new life in Christ Jesus. This call has been unheard except for a few fundamentalist preachers who recognize this deteriorating situation for what it was and spoke up. Society's present state proves that the Gospel must include both the love of Christ and the judgment of God against sin.

Before we cast the first stone, however, we must remember that we are all tempted. And we all struggle as we come to the point of commiting sin or resisting temptation. We must make a conscious effort to say "no" to sin. We should also recognize it is the power of the Holy Spirit that helps us to resist. We are all unworthy of the grace offered to us by a loving Heavenly Father.

To recover the ground we have lost, to revive our calling and to pluck sinners from the hand of Satan, we must learn to protect our minds and the minds of our children from society's sexual consensus. We must remember it is by the grace of God that we are His. Our compassion must be rekindled to share both the love of Christ and God's judgment against sin just as the compassion of Christ saved us from punishment.

In counseling patients with sexual questions or problems, I have found almost all of the techniques taught in medical schools to be worthless, primarily because they support the use of sex for pleasure. Deprogramming the mind, understanding the messages that have been instilled through the media is the first step; and simplicity is the key.

I have used three, simple titles to help patients understand the perversions of sexuality: sex for sale, sex for pleasure, and sex for self.

SEX FOR SALE

Selling all types of products is their aim; through sexually suggestive advertising, their game. The social engineers of the world have picked the most powerful tools to change the hearts and minds of the American public — the tools of education, public school curricula, entertainment and advertising.

Advertisers have two directives in creating visual advertisements — to educate about their product and to create a desire for that product. Text and spoken word give specific product claims, availabilty, quantity, usage, quality, ability, etc. The visual qualities of the product, the props, and the people within an advertisement, along with the text, create in the consumer a desire to obtain that product over other competitive products.

Many studies show the power of visual stimuli in altering behavior and passing on information. The saying, "A picture is worth a thousand words," is very true, encouraging advertisers to sell by visual desire instead of factual comparisons of products. Though the action of the pictorial advertisement may be subtle, the resulting change in behavior proves the effectiveness of this approach.

How many times have you stopped to look at products that have the simple four-letter word over them, marked SALE? How many men do double-takes when they see a billboard sign with a shiny new car that has a barely clothed model sitting on top of it? Is he really "checking-out" the car with that second look? Have you ever, when watching television, seen a commercial with a cold, wet, sparkling soft-drink, and then realized you were thirsty enough to go get a drink, possibly even the same soft-drink?

What we see triggers us to desire a product and to accept the world's view of that product. Most producers use sexually suggestive models, actions, words, or inflection to create a desire for their product. Wine producers show beautiful couples, dressed for seduction, sipping their product with pursed lips. After tasting the wine, they sigh and smile as if in ecstasy. Canned fruit products, not usually consumed at romantic times, use a couple dressed in evening wear, touching and caressing each other while eating canned peaches, showing sensual lips and suggestive movements that all could be occurring, except for the formal dress, in a private bedroom.

Products that have sexual connotations, such as make-up, jewelry, lipstick, clothing, underwear and shoes, are advertised with the sexiest actions, postures, clothing, and sounds possible. Even non-sexual products, such as toothpaste, soft-drinks, cars, food products and cigarettes show how their products are able to improve the user's sexual attractiveness to the opposite sex.

This sexual harassment by advertising slowly dulls our sensitivity to these open sexual displays, allows sex to become a bought and sold commodity, suggests the appropriateness of open sexual display and promotes sex as the primary determinant of good and bad products, services and actions. When we watch advertisements use these specific tactics every day, we find our perception of normal sexual behavior becomes twisted to conform with the world's values.

Advertisers, marketers and retailers have used the lure of sensuality to create a desire in the buyer for many different products. Besides using sex as a selling point, they have incorporated the two other areas of temptation, lust of the eyes and the pride of life to their monetary advantage. The visual beauty of the product, enhanced by the model, instills in us a want even if there is no practical reason to buy the product. This is a form of lust of the eyes. The promise of a product that we will have success, power, stature, love, and money makes us believe the product will enhance our image. This is a form of pride of life.

The positive aspects of sex within marriage have been exchanged by the world to suggest that sex is for sale and that it is something we all need lots of. This materialistic perversion suggests sex is not rare, saved for that special person who will give himself/herself totally and only to you. Instead, sex is for pleasure, for everyone to share, to be tried out, to be sold for a date, to get as much as you can. That sex is for sale makes it awfully cheap.

God's principles are broken by following the world's philosophy of sex for sale; and when God's principles are violated, sinners are hurt.

SEX FOR SELF

The "me" generation has left indelible scars on the face of our society. Families are no longer important to many persons; and success, careers, personal comfort, material possessions are now what is essential. Children are no longer a blessing from the Lord, but a burden, an unwanted pregnancy, a tax deduction, a daily trip to the "day-care center." People have changed their expectations about life and how it should be lived. Work must be endured, so that we can party at night, relax on weekends, and play on vacations. "Eat, drink, and be sexual" is the unspoken motto of the world.

The promotion of self tempts the sin nature to be prideful, always looking to help number one, using any means to climb on top of others. Sex is for self-stimulation, self-gratification, personal enjoyment and, yes, if your sexual partner had a good time, then all is well. Sex books and manuals tout more gratification and more pleasure for those who read these powerful pages. Your "lovers" will desire to be with you more, and you will have mystical sexual powers over them. Special devices are created and sold to increase the pleasure of sexual relations.

The world feeds those who hunger after sin with the bread of pleasure and the milk of pride. And, according to God's principles, pride comes before the fall.

SEX FOR PLEASURE

Sexual relationships are pleasurable, whether they occur within or outside of marriage. Sexual pleasure within marriage is a beautiful bonus to the real reasons for sex, that of building oneness in marriage, promoting love and trust and procreating. Committed married partners would probably still have sexual relations even if it were unpleasant as long as it brought union to the marriage and created children.

Pleasure becomes the world's primary goal for a sexual relationship, dispelling the need for commitment, trust and fidelity. Seeking after pleasure is life's highest aim. Personal pleasure and orgasm become the reason for sex, for a relationship, for existence.

But seeking after pleasure is an unending spiral. Those who seek after money know that it cannot buy happiness and the appetite for more money consistently outgrows what is received. The same is true with such pleasures as sex. The appetite for sex consistently grows more rapidly than the ability to quench that appetite. An individual can starve to death if his appetite grows too big.

The world's call for pleasure only debases the marriage relationship, children, and God's principles for proper use. God's punishment for sex abuse is an unquenchable desire.

NON-JUDGMENTALISM

One of the most blaring hypocrisies that I learned in medical school is the attitude of non-judgmentalism. We are taught not to judge people's actions, sexually, as there is no

Plague in Our Midst

right and wrong in this area. However, we are taught to teach our patients that certain behaviors are unhealthy, such as smoking, overeating, and driving without a seatbelt. We teach preventative health in these areas, but we were taught that prevention in the sexual areas is "judgmental."

I have long since decided that telling my patients the truth, the biblical principles about sexuality, was by far the best, most helpful way to counsel. The Bible hasn't been wrong yet.

Here is an example of how a physician uses "medically-acceptable," non-judgmental therapy with a client.

In a large town, a male client came to his physician because he was having impotence problems with his wife. This man admitted to frequently and continually using hardcore pornography, prostitutes, masturbation and had even attended a gay bathhouse. He was able in each of these situations to complete the act but when he got home was unable to get enough stimulation. The physician using standard, non-judgmental therapy suggested the following:

Use the pornography closer to the time of having relations with your wife. Try to use prostitutes and self-stimulation less so that you will have more sexual energy when you see your wife. If your impotence continues, there may be a need for antidepressants that can help your situation. After a trial time of six months, if things do not improve sexually with your wife, you may want to consider another partner.

All health professionals are trained to counsel their clients in this non-judgmental way, never suggesting a certain pattern of behavior is wrong especially when it comes to sexual intercourse. The guilt and depression, the inability to ask forgiveness from his wife and his unwillingness to stop these extrememly vile behaviors are the major source of this man's problem; but the physician will never mention any of this. The proper therapy, stopping all illicit behaviors, asking for forgiveness from the wife and dealing with his guilt and depression are considered "judgmental therapy" and would be likened to malpractice.

Part of our medical school curriculum included the viewing of "hard-core" pornography to "desensitize" physicians to perverted sexual relationships. This practice is supposed to promote long-term professional relationships and to encourage open communication of problems. Few physicians, after viewing these films, are shocked by what their patients tell them.

Sexual counselors encourage experimentation with other forms of intercourse or with different partners to "improve sexual function" or to cure impotence. Feelings are explored, sensations are promoted, anger and guilt are released so that the ultimate act, that of intercourse, can be accomplished without any hindrances. A counselor who judges certain sexual behaviors as unhealthy does not promote the patient's well-being — in the world's eyes.

Marriage counselors are not supposed to cast blame or to work out problems but to be non-judgmental and to facilitate discussion. Some counselors open their client sessions by stating, "I am not here to heal your marriage, but to make sure each of you finds the happiest and best solution for your problem." In their opinion divorce is always an option.

All of these professionals receive money from clients for advice as to the best treatment or the best course of action. What intelligent physician would not tell the patient to stop smoking before lung disease is detected? Professionals are paid to judge what is best for the client and that includes values, principles and relationships. It must include sexuality.

Non-judgmentalism has worked effectively to instill the open sexual values into the minds and hearts of intellectuals within the health care and educational fields. But it is encouraging the continued slide toward hedonism because it refuses to condemn any and all vile behaviors.

TREATMENT OF THE MIND

The sin sickness that has invaded the American mind has done great damage to the personal, sprirtual, and

Plague in Our Midst

sexual lives of its people. Minds and hearts today are filled with perverse images and uncontrollable desires for sexual relationships that are risky, promiscuous and dangerous.

Analogies are a favorite teaching tool of mine, often shedding understanding on difficult areas of human physiology. This "perverse mind," filled with images of self-centered sexuality, is similar to drugs or alcohol. When too much of the drug has been taken, the senses are dulled, the mind is overly happy, and the thoughts are confused. Similar malfunctioning occurs when the mind is filled with thoughts of promiscuous sexual experiences. The conscience is dulled to sin, the mind is hooked on pleasure and proper thinking about consequences is confused.

The treatment is to remove the confusing agent. Stopping the drug or alcohol will produce rapid restoration of the original mind. Removal of perverse sexual thoughts from the mind is a slow, disciplined process of mental and spiritual renewal, but it must be accomplished before there can be restoration.

For patients who have problems with sexual thoughts or who are caught up into the promiscuous mindset of the world, I often prescribe "mind renewal" from Ephesians chapter four. Retrain your mind to keenly discern temptations, the world's images of sex for sale, for self, for pleasure, and then shut your mind to this stimulation. I tell them that when these images of "sinful sex" come into their mind, images they remember from previous experiences or pictures they've seen, they must suppress them and push these perversions out of conscious thought by filling the mind with "good, spiritual things."

Exercising the Spirit within us keeps us strong and able to resist the desires of the flesh. Prayer and study of the Scripture on a daily schedule sustains a growing communion with our Lord and strengthens the "right" desires in our heart and right thoughts in our minds.

Avoiding places, persons or situations that are often associated with promiscuous sexuality is wise if we want to prevent our falling into temptation. The process of mental renewal must be accompanied by patience, as removal of these images takes months to years.

Our spiritual responsibility is to renew our minds, our desires, our sexual attitudes so that they will be aligned with the ideals of Scripture and so that our thoughts and actions will be pleasing to God. We are also responsible for shaping the minds of our children through Scripture and for giving them the values upon which they will build their sexual attitudes.

CHAPTER FIVE
SEX EDUCATION AND SCRIPTURAL PRINCIPLES

    Parents always seem to feel that sex education is either God-sent or Satan-delivered for their children. Some see knowledge as the only reasonable way to give their children the proper tools for handling difficult sexual decisions. Others see children taught to beget other children, long before they are responsible and mature enough to handle the situation.

    From a strictly medical standpoint, I always seem to deal with the failures, those who were taught but would not listen. I deal with those young women who became pregnant or the young men with venereal disease.

    I routinely ask these young people if they have received sex education. More than 90 percent have said yes. But when I ask them about using birth control, I often hear this reply: "I really wanted to learn about sex, but could care less about birth control. Now I wish I had listened."

Here is a personal story of a young lady who ended up in a local maternity program. Her story is rather typical, similar to the 25 percent of all young women who will become pregnant before marriage.

Charlene was excited about school. She was entering seventh grade, moving to a new building next to the high school and eating with the high school classes. She was especially anxious about health class, where she was told by peers that "sex" was being taught. Her physical maturity was on par with some of the older freshmen, yet she was socially very immature. She had been allowed to date only the last year and only to school functions. As third period drew closer, Charlene grew more excited.

The first few class periods in health were not that exciting. In the second week they talked about reproduction, the sperm and the egg, fertilization, implantation and pregnancy. In the third and fourth weeks, they started to talk about intrapersonal relationships, the heavy term for dates. Much of what was taught revolved around normal feelings, the lusts, the drives and desires that teens have. As well, they described intercourse during dates, premarital sex, and homosexual feelings and sex.

The teacher never talked about values in these discussions and often asked, "How do you feel about this?" Birth control was treated as a way of avoiding pregnancy, especially if the urge was overpowering. Abstinence was not promoted as a means of birth control but just as a side thought. Marriage was something that happened when two individuals loved each other as confirmed by their sexual compatibility and their ability to stimulate each other.

As with any immature young lady, the urge was stronger than the intellectual reasons for restraint. On some of her dates, Charlene was very open to sexual experimentation, believing that pregnancy would not happen to her. She had three boy friends and intercourse five times. Six months after starting seventh grade, she withdrew to enroll in an unwed maternity program in a distant city.

Was Charlene helped by her sex education program?

FAILURE OF SEX EDUCATION

Public schools cannot be trusted to teach Christ-centered sexual attitudes, or to teach a fair and balanced approach to human sexuality. Why? Their predominant philosophy, humanism, promotes promiscuous sexuality. Humanism expresses itself in the minds and curricula of educators, in non-judgementalism of deviant forms of sexuality, in promotion of promiscuity by teaching about intercourse and in teaching immature adults how to "beat the system" by using birth control. All this contributes to a continuous progression toward more open sexuality.

The term "sex education" provokes fear and anger in the hearts of many Christian parents, and rightfully so. Some schools teach valueless rehearsals of sexual intercourse where marriage is one of a number of acceptable lifestyles. School officials believe that children cannot develop sexual self-control and they offer no alternatives to promiscuity besides birth control as protection from pregnancy. Others teach situational ethics concerning sexual relationships, pregnancy and promiscuity that are devoid of any and all biblical values. Modern interpretation of the Constitution suggests that public schools and religious values concerning sex must be separated for the safety of the children.

Teaching pre-adolescent and early adolescent children about intercourse is something like teaching a bank robber about the alarm system, the safe, the safety deposit boxes and the exits but warning him not to get caught. No proof can be mustered to show that this type of sex education has helped reduce pregnancy rates, venereal disease or abortion. In fact, our teen pregnancy rate is twice that of other "civilized countries" that offer sex education to their children.

What are we doing wrong? Our errors — self-indulgence, non-judgemental attitudes, freedom from responsibility, and the utter disregard of societal values — are deep-seated in the basic philosophies of the world. These philosophies led to confused, experimental sex education curricula that negatively affect the sexual behavior of teens. Many of our worst social problems — abortion, teen pregnancy, AIDS and venereal disease — have been perpetuated through these classes and the "situational" values taught in them.

Where do these sex education classes miss the mark? Many school programs teach the wrong concepts for specific age and grade level. Teaching an immature sixth or seventh grader about intercourse is like teaching a three-or four-year-old to type before he can read.

Most public school sex education programs are devoid of values and principles concerning the "wrongness" or "rightness" of birth control, abortion, intercourse and other topics. All scriptural teaching underlines the "wrongness" of sin and the "rightness" of godly living.

Few programs discuss the role of sexuality within a permanent male-female relationship, how it should be used and what constitutes abnormal or abusive sexuality. Scripture clearly discusses sexuality within the self-sacrificial, loving, nurturing confines of marriage.

In the past, most programs have neglected to discuss responsibility as an essential element in any consideration of sexual intercourse. Fortunately, many programs have since added this particular area, but much of the damage has already been done. Teaching personal responsibility to immature children while tempting them with the "bare essentials" of sex leads to desire without restraint.

Birth control and thus intercourse is encouraged as normal behavior. Preventing pregnancy becomes the primary goal of a sexual relationship. The promoting of proper sexual behavior, self-control and chastity — the biblical mandates — has no place.

Abstinence prior to marriage is the most important, most effective means of birth control. It eliminates venereal disease and promotes healthy adult sexuality within marriage. Yet most schools barely mention this concept or suggest its value because teachers sense that most students will inevitably have sex.

The best way to prevent someone from becoming "hooked" on the pleasurable aspects of smoking, drinking, drugs and sex is to not have them start. The most important problem with most programs is the lack of a strong abstinence message — SAY NO TO SEX, SAY YES TO ABSTINENCE.

Most Christian parents rightfully object to the exposure of their children to these valueless philosophies. The "world" is given an open door to creep into the minds and hearts of youngsters exposed to sex education in the public schools. The immaturity and gullibility of children who are just formulating their own value structure make them more susceptible to the compromise of their proper beliefs by this exposure.

KNOWLEDGE AND COMPARISON

Was Charlene better off knowing about sexuality, intercourse, birth control, abstinence and the many other concepts of sexuality? Are people in general better off because they know the sex life of their neighbors, their heroes, their society? Has this increase in knowledge about sexual function been a help or hindrance to people today?

Sexuality has always been an extremely private act between two persons who have committed themselves through marriage to a lifetime of intimacy and sharing. Scripture supports this extremely "private" view of sex and castigates those who make public use of sexual display in entertainment, advertising and pornography.

Now most persons do know how other people have sex, the whys, whens, and the wheres. It is common knowledge about the number of times couples are to have intimacy, what types of birth control are used, what positions are most stimulating. And the information goes on and on. Sex education courses add to this public display of sexual intimacy.

Kelly and Caron were both raised in very strict, Christian homes. No dating was allowed until age 18 and then only with a chaperone. Both were sent to the same Christian college because of the strictness of the atmosphere. Neither had sex education courses or any exposure to pornography and very little exposure to magazines and television. Prior to their wedding, both parents sat down with their young adult and discussed concepts of marriage, homemaking and sexuality.

Their wedding night came and went. Both were very satisfied with the beginning of a sexual relationship that by public standards was an absolute disaster. Intercourse had not been seriously attempted, yet they were still very satisfied just spending time together, sharing themselves, getting to know and trust each other more.

If this couple were to have been grounded in the usual knowledge of our culture, their sex life would have been a flat failure and their marriage doomed to die. Thank God, they did not know what they supposedly were missing. Kelly and Caron were very satisfied, not because they performed as well as expected, but because they had given themselves completely and tenderly to one another. They were fortunate to have light baggage, little sexual imagery and training from the world's view of sexuality.

The more public sex becomes, the more mental baggage our young persons take into a relationship. They believe that climax is the purpose of sex, not the reward. They have mental pictures of the perfect bodies seen in extremely provocative poses in pornography, and they expect their relationship to be equally as perfect and provocative. They know how they must perform if they are to be "great lovers" as the world would describe them. There is a constant comparison of notes, of techniques, of positions so that lovemaking can be improved.

Public knowledge about sexual functioning and comparisons of sexual relationships distorts the purpose of sexuality in a relationship. Sexual intimacy was designed by

God to allow oneness, sharing, tenderness, caring, warmth and love to be shown one to another. Sexual climax is a very brief, pleasurable moment that passes sperm from male to female, allowing for procreation to occur. It is not the sole purpose nor the most important part of sex within a marriage relationship.

Sex education courses that publicize knowledge about sexuality serve to promote the sex for self, sex for pleasure principles by comparing one couple's sex life to another's. Sex education within the Christian home — that promotes the private, intimate aspects of the sexual relationship, that promotes abstinence until marriage and suggests that love, intimacy, and sharing are more important than climax — will greatly serve to promote healthy sexual attitudes in our children.

REDEFINING SEX EDUCATION

For most school systems, sex education is defined as a "how to" course — how to have intercourse, how to take birth control, how to seek abortions, how not to judge others for their sexual behaviors and attitudes and how not to tell your parents. Some school systems attempt to depict sexual intercourse in marriage as the most appropriate place for this behavior, yet do not judge homosexual, premarital or extra-marital intercourse. These double standards only serve to confuse the children they are trying to educate.

As suggested above, the concept of sex education must be redefined for consumption by the Christian family. Sex education for the Christian family must be distinctively different, based on a solid biblical foundation and filled with honesty and knowledge about the problems that are present in our society. It must support the privacy, purity and uniqueness of the sex life for any married couple, while refraining from the comparisons and valueless knowledge that fills the mind with detracting ideas.

"My son, keep your father's commands and do not

forsake your mother's teaching. Bind them upon your heart forever; fasten them around your neck. When you walk, they will guide you; when you sleep, they will watch over you; when you awake, they will speak to you. For these commands are a lamp, this teaching is a light, and the corrections of discipline are the way of life, keeping you from the immoral woman .... Proverbs 6:20-24 (NIV)

The family is the only appropriate place for education concerning sexual attitudes and function; and the schools, including Christian day schools, are no substitute. Parents are to be active role models for their children as well as teachers of the biblical principles of male-female relationships. Unless children see the consistency of parental role models on a daily basis, they may confuse normal sexual attitudes with the loose sexual behavior they see in the media or in other families. The basis of a scriptural marital and sexual relationship is the love, trust and self-sacrifice shown through observation of non-verbal communication and affection. Children cannot learn this from a book or lecture.

Sexual attitude education must start young. The concepts must be appropriate to the age and must be taught with sensitivity to the individual's needs, understanding and maturity. A first grader obviously should not be taught about the act of intercourse, but may be taught about marriage, why people get married, and what the scriptural responsibilities of marriage are. Between the ages of 10 and 12, open discussion about feelings, lusts, hormones, body changes and the consequences of premature sexual intercourse are appropriate for most. Young adults in their late teens or early twenties should be familiarized with more of the concepts of sexual intercourse within marriage and proper self-care and health-care, especially if they are nearing a marriage relationship themselves.

Christian individuals and the church should remain firm in their support of sex education through God's educational unit, the family. Private Christian schools should also be willing to help parents learn about the biblical basis of sexuality, methods of instruction, age appropriate concepts, role-modeling, and how to answer difficult sexual questions.

Redefining and redirecting sex education is a large task, but one the Christian community needs to accomplish if we are to be salt for a dying world.

SCRIPTURAL PRINCIPLES FOR SEX EDUCATION

Parents are blessed with the most wonderful, fulfilling, and precious of all earthly gifts — their children. They are also charged with the solemn responsibility to raise those children "in the nurture and admonition of the Lord."

Instruction of sexual attitudes and function has long been a difficult area of discussion in the Christian home for a wide variety of reasons. Christian parents may not want to be seen as "immoral" persons, possessing knowledge and understanding of the topic of sexuality. They hide the image of being "sexually informed" to preserve the illusion they are pure and untarnished by the ways of the world. Many Christian parents from godly families have not been exposed to sexual attitudes and function, with the exception of basic scriptural references to marriage and temptation. Misinformation and myths that sexual sins cause bizarre diseases have been passed through generations to deter young adults from sexual promiscuity. As a result, they've relayed a negative attitude toward all sexual teachings.

One morning I came into the office and my secretary stopped me, warning me that three messages were on my door, all from the same mother. When I returned the call, I found a distraught mother who was seeking advice on how to handle her son's habit of masturbation.

This mother had consulted friends and a pastor in the area who all suggested telling her son myths about blindness, venereal disease and future sexual problems. She had felt uncomfortable with this off-the-cuff advice and wanted a medical opinion from a Christian physician. It had been three days since she had accidentally walked in on her adolescent son who was stimulating himself.

My suggestions were simple. No diseases are contracted through masturbation, and misinforming him about these would have been wrong. However, he needs to know that repeated stimulation could make premature ejaculation a problem in marriage. Her positive encouragement using truthful information, not myths to scare him into stopping, would probably accomplish the desired result, and help her to build communication with her son.

From a spiritual standpoint those who arouse themselves visualize stimulating and pornographic images. This is the "lust of the flesh" decried as sin in Scripture. As this young man was born-again, praying with him and showing him the specific Scriptures that denounce these lusts would allow the Holy Spirit to convict and protect from temptation. Biblically the habit does not glorify God in our lives.

A few weeks later, this mother stopped me at church with some good news. The young man had greatly reduced his habit. He usually felt strong enough to resist when temptations aroused him. The mother admitted, as I had suggested, that sometimes you give in when you are trying to break a difficult and addictive habit such as masturbation. But minor setbacks should not destroy the overall progess made in breaking the habit.

Sure enough, he had been open and willing to communicate with his mother about a number of other problems. Their relationship had never been better.

We no longer have the luxury of hiding from these topics of sexuality. Our children are demanding answers to difficult questions. They are being tempted to partake of forbidden fruits. They are crying for information, openness and communication from parents. We must respond with knowledge, not myths; with positiveness, not shame; with information, not hearsay; all based on the principles and values of Scripture.

ATTITUDES AND PRINCIPLES

What drives us to action? How do we make decisions about our behavior toward our family, our friends, our community? What shapes the way we think and gives us ready comparisons for reference? What are the building blocks for human behavior?

It often baffles me when a patient comes into the office, confesses that he "missed his medication" and then justifies both the reasons and the consequences with "excuses." If I could invent some pill to ensure that patients would faithfully take their treatments as prescribed, I could avert untold suffering and have untold millions of dollars fall into my bank account. Regulating healthy behavior would be almost heaven for all physicians.

Understanding behavior, thoughts, principles, values, memories and experiences that drive behaviors into actions, have been attempted since early biblical times. When it comes to sexuality, we need to shape, reform, or reconstruct these parts of behavior before attitudes become promiscuous actions. In fact, it is the primary purpose of this book to change the way we think about sexuality, about open sexual displays and about the way we train our children. We cannot change sexual behaviors until we change sexual attitudes.

Attitudes consist of knowledge, principles, values, ideas, memories, and feelings about any subject area. Our attitudes give the mental direction and content to behavior and the thoughts leading to action. Sexual attitudes likewise govern our sexual functioning as adolescents or adults.

Could you imagine the problems if you gave an immature adolescent the keys to the car, money for gasoline, and told him, "There are no rules to driving. Just try not to hurt someone." He would do just that! Tire tracks across the lawn, mailboxes smashed, cars dented and persons injured or killed are all the probable results of irresponsibility without the restraints of laws and principles.

The same is true for sexual behavior. The world says, "Do anything, try anything, just don't hurt the other person."

That is why parents must take great care and effort to ground their children in a thorough understanding of the scriptural attitudes of sexuality.

Here is a true story about principles.

At 19, Mary Sue was on her own. Two weeks before, her parents were tragically killed in an automobile crash. Her boyfriend Craig was a great comfort to her during this extremely difficult time in her life. They had been planning to tell their parents at Easter of their plans to be married when school was finished. In the midst of her non-stop tears, Mary Sue could hear her father saying, "Be faithful 'till the end, and you will not be disappointed."

The desire was overwhelming to jump into bed with Craig, to solidify that union, to be comforted, held and loved. Yet the principles that Mary Sue saw in her father and mother were so real, they smothered the desire for easy sex. They had taught her the scriptural principles that waiting sexually would bring blessing to a marriage.

She and Craig did not betray their parents' teachings and were married one year later. They both completed their college degrees with honors; and they loved, respected, and trusted each other more than when tragedy had tempted them. There would be no guilt in their marriage, no guilt of failure to please their parents, no guilt of succumbing to sexual temptation, no guilt of sin.

Each of us desires to instill in our children the ability to make proper, God-honoring decisions. We encourage them and pray that they will make few mistakes. It is impossible to regulate their experiences, memories and ideas. Our impact comes in teaching principles and values that build the important foundation upon which all their behavior is formed.

PRINCIPLES OF SEXUALITY

As with all of God's eternal truths, purity and simplicity will draw each of us through the Holy Spirit to an understanding of God's purpose for our lives. Scriptural principles are almost too simple for us to believe realistic, yet when we put them into practice we find they yield profound benefits that only the faithful follower will comprehend.

Scripture speaks firmly, purely and simply on all aspects of human sexuality. What are these simple principles that will give the one who follows them great personal reward? How can negative principles be so positive? What is the best way to pass these along to our children?

In my discussions of sexuality with patients, I use the following scriptural principles as a simple, three-point outline in understanding sexual attitudes. There are other principles that pertain to sexuality, but these three are the most important in teaching others — or our children: –

FIRST, PROMISCUOUS SEXUALITY IS SIN; THEREFORE, BE OBEDIENT.

God promises retribution and judgment on those who commit adultery or fornication. Diseases and plagues will come upon those who spurn God's commands. Personal and family problems will follow those who defile the marriage bed. Sexual sin in individuals will bring reproach upon the society that tolerates their vile behavior.

God promises retribution for breaking His laws and blessings for keeping his laws.

For every negative command in Scripture, there is always a positive reward, a blessing from God that is hidden and promised for those who faithfully uphold His Word. We often dwell upon restrictions placed upon us by Scripture instead of seeing the potential God has designed within creation for our good, our pleasure an our edification. Sexuality is a beautiful, God-designed blessing if we are only wise enough to forego temporal satisfaction for marital bliss and eternal rewards.

SECOND, YOUR BODY BELONGS TO YOUR MATE; THEREFORE, SACRIFICE YOURSELF.

There is no greater act of giving love, of self-sacrificial commitment between two persons who desire a lifetime of happiness, than the giving of themselves completely, purely and wholly to the other in sexual communion. To give away your body in promiscuous experimentation prior to marriage is similar to giving your wife to another man during marriage. Scripture states that your body belongs to your mate whether before or after marriage. It is the temple of God to be sacrificially kept pure for the marital partner.

Sexuality is a private act between two married people. It should be special, saved only for the spouse. Sex does not build love and trust, a hope that spurs many a teen woman to give her body to a man in exchange for love. Love and trust build the sexual relationship. Many sad testimonies have been given about a growing, beautiful premarital relationship destroyed by the premature giving in to each other sexually.

THIRD, WAITING BRINGS GREAT REWARDS;THEREFORE LIVE BY FAITH

There is always a choice between faith and sin. Faith is trusting in God's commands and waiting for God's blessing. Sin is living for the momentary pleasure and not waiting to fulfill an urge, a desire, a lust. All of life is either faithful decisions leading to maturity, reward, and faith or sinful decisions leading to pain, reproach and addiction to pleasure.

Obedience to God's laws, self-sacrificial waiting for the marriage partner and faith built through patience, these are the principles of Scripture that build proper sexual attitudes. These are the principles we need to share with our children so they "will not depart" from behavior that pleases our Father.

CHAPTER SIX
Teaching Children About Sexual Attitudes

The ability of children to learn is amazing. I'm often humbled by how quickly our seven-year-old daughter learns to calculate a math problem or the meaning of a new word or how to beat me at a video game. Just last year, our two-year-old was barely uttering an understandable sentence; now he "preaches" during his dinner-time prayer.

Seeing the rapid intellectual growth of my pediatric patients is an ever-present reminder of how little time we have to teach our children the concepts and skills they will use as adults. Children consistently grow faster than our motivation or ability to train them does.

So training their sexual attitudes should begin at a very early age. It normally begins from the time a one- or two-year-old child sees and understands the physical differences between mother and father, brothers and sisters. It continues when he understands the difference between "Mega-man" and "Wonder-woman" on the Saturday morning cartoons. It is always being shaped and redefined by new images and new relationships from pre-school days through adulthood.

The central, reoccurring themes — the scriptural principles — I often share with patients give a firm foundation for discussions of these sexual attitudes. As described before, these principles are obedience, self-sacrifice and faith. Obedience corresponds to following God's commands, reaping the blessings and avoiding the punishments. It is a self-sacrificial act to protect and keep pure the body that does not belong to you but belongs to your mate. Faith is built up by refusing to succumb to temporal temptations and by waiting for the promised rewards of obedience. Using these principles as a central outline will make this difficult task of teaching our children about sex a much easier and more scripturally oriented process.

But teaching children about sexual attitudes is more than giving them the abstract principles of Scripture. Children need concrete examples of these important lifestyle concepts. Showing them how to act, what to say, what pleases God, and what is worldly enticement, is essential. Consistently discussing these concepts as our children become involved in situations, or as they see others making sexually based decisions, is wise. Never neglect the power of example. Showing our children how to live, and not just telling them, is important.

Entire books have been written on the topic of teaching sexuality to children. Many have excellent approaches and worthwhile information. But, the aim of this book will be to teach the simple, sufficient scriptural principles of sexuality. Simplification improves memory of the principles and thus makes these concepts more applicable. When decisions arise, there are fewer options to be considered. Simplification keeps Scripture as the foundation for all of sexuality, the important position it should hold.

Our discussion of these principles will be divided into

four age groups: pre-school, early school age, adolescent, and pre-marriage groups. As we age, our ability to understand more and more abstract concepts matures; and these differences in our ability to learn make many concepts appropriate for only certain age groups.

Though neglected in most sex-education curricula, the pre-school age group is the age to begin teaching about sexual differences and how they apply to obedience, self-sacrifice and faith.

PRE-SCHOOL LEVEL — AGES 3 TO 6

A kindergarten teacher finished reading the story of the "Three Little Pigs" and then asked her group of four-and five-year-olds some questions.

"Was the wolf in the story a boy-wolf or a girl-wolf?" All of the children raised their hands for "boy-wolf."

"Why do you think he was a boy?"

"He was strong and mean," said one boy.

"He wore suspenders and jeans," said another boy.

"Girls don't have hairy chins," said one girl indignantly. Even four-and five-year-old children have mental images of what a boy is and what a girl is. They know that clothing, facial appearance, hair, voices, actions, are all points of differentiation between the sexes. They have discovered these characteristics through observing family, friends, television, pictures and simply by comparing people in their world. It is a natural learning process that occurs normally with little parental input.

Yet, understanding gender is considered a developmental task, an important building-block of normal maturation. Gender, or sexual identity, builds individual self-esteem in your children as they identify with a parent of the same sex and by understanding their place in the family. They build a gender identity through friendships with friends of the same gender. We all grow up wanting to fit into the world around us.

How exactly do we teach our children about sexual attitudes? Do we have "home sex school" or do we supplement public school texts with family "couch" talks?

My suggestion is to think of every moment with your children as a teaching moment. Opportunity after opportunity will arise in conversation between you and with other people (or when viewing or reading some piece of media) that will present positive or negative images of sexuality to your children. At once is the best time to correct or reinforce that image before it fades from their memory.

Here are some practical thoughts about discussing sexuality. When you are watching TV with the kids and you see a "sexual" situation, you can discuss the content of the scene. Does it portray a woman as a beautiful body only, a hard-working supermom or a wonderful creation of God? Does it portray men as a nude upper torso, a brilliant executive making decisions or a spiritual leader in the home?

Watching how your kids play — the characters, the content, the imagination — gives you feedback about the roles they are imitating. It tells you what characteristics they attribute to men and women.

Communicating with your children, as the important persons they are, builds their self-esteem. Don't always be harsh, measuring their thoughts or actions with a judging attitude. Talk with your children about the motives behind their actions. This causes them to think and give reasons for their behavior. It reminds them they are accountable for their actions.

Our spiritual responsibility as parents is two-fold. First, we are to be a discipler, one who teaches biblical principles for living. Second, is to be an encourager, one who provides the motivation and the strength to follow our lead. Positive encouragement to follow and to be obedient to God's principles is the most productive task of parenting.

Most parents realize that trying to teach abstract concepts to pre-school children is virtually useless. Experts in child development suggest using "concrete" concepts — objects, actions and people — to illustrate a point. Pre-schoolers do this naturally, comparing one person to another, one object to another, to see how they are different. We need to begin teaching our children about sexual attitudes by using these concrete concepts, such as differences in physical appearance and difference in roles and behaviors.

PHYSICAL DIFFERENCES

The most easily noticed sexual differences are physical: fathers are often taller and stronger than mothers and have shorter hair; mothers are shorter, softer and have longer hair. It becomes a routine task for younger children to mentally compare things and to learn from the differences they detect. Talking about these differences will refine a pre-schooler's power of observation and point out qualities to look for.

The major physical difference between men and women, that even a three-year-old can understand, is that women bear children and men cannot. Pre-schoolers should be told of the need for two people, a married couple, to be present before a "mommy" can have children. This initiates an understanding of marriage, the necessity for a loving relationship to be established before children are born. An abstract concept that "strikes home" for many children is that they are a product of mommy's and daddy's "love." This is an adequate way for pre-schoolers to be introduced to the concept of sexual relations and proves to be a self-esteem building idea for the child.

Pre-school children are always exploring their environment through their concrete senses of sight, hearing, touch, smell, and feeling. Introducing them to the many physical things that make mommies and daddies brings clarity to differences in roles, actions and behaviors. What clothing would a daddy wear? Are daddies stronger than mommies? What tools or objects does a mommy use? What things in the house or yard does mommy take care of, and what things does daddy take care of?

Comparisons of specific body characteristics allow the child to compare similarities and differences between himself or herself and mother or father. Acting out some of these gender differences, such a mother acting like a father, can be a learning experience for both parent and child. This is called role reversal and highlights characteristics that are different.

Play can be an excellent reinforcer of gender differences. "I am stronger, bigger and meaner than you, so I will be the daddy." The tender, caring, rocking motions of a mother holding her child are commonly imitated behaviors for pre-school girls and occasionally boys.

Obedience is the obvious and essential scriptural concept to teach in this age group. But teaching obedience by punishment only is not scriptural. God promises blessings for those who willingly obey and punishment for those who willingly disobey. So we must also balance our discipline, reward our children for their rapid and willing completion of a task and depriving or spanking them for severe disobedience that could lead to harm.

Parents can be excellent examples of obedience as well as personal demonstrations of promised spiritual rewards. Being obedient in praying for others and then receiving God's perfect answers as a consequence will allow children to see God's blessing in obedience. Fathers who faithfully and obediently provide for their families are fulfilling God's design and will be blessed for their hard work. Mothers who willingly and lovingly care for their family's needs, whether inside or outside the home, will also receive God's blessing for obedience. Children who obey their parents are blessed with respect, love and little "painful" discipline. There are many other practical, everyday situations where obedience brings blessing and discussing these with your children will continue to engrain these concepts in their lives.

God designed the physical and emotional differences

Plague in Our Midst

between men and women to fit different purposes, to fulfill different roles. These created differences make men and women perfect companions for one another, each completing what the other lacked, each helping where the other is unable, each being fruitful where one alone is not enough.

DIFFERENCES IN ROLES

What are the real roles for men and women in our society? It seems like the world has redesigned the traditional roles of men and women, stripping each of their God-given uniqueness so each may strive for a single "uni-sex" identity. Through this redefinition, the value of marriage, family and especially children has been reduced.

The change in roles creates tremendous and unnecessary stresses on the minds of so many people. Psychiatrists, psychologists, and even I in my own family practice — we all find patients filling the waiting room with stress-related physical and emotional problems. Burn-out syndrome, two-career marriages, dysfunctional communication are all aggravated by the competition of men against women for careers, jobs, promotions, positions and money.

This results in damage to our children who are confused about which parent they are to imitate and to which gender they belong. Confusion in this area will make it difficult for them to model one specific pattern of gender behavior and may lead to damaged self-esteem and social withdrawal.

Where do we begin to teach real, biblical male and female roles to our children? Here are some thoughts.

In obedience to Scripture, young people leave their parents, marry, and live together as commanded by the Lord:

"For this reason a man will leave his father and mother and be united to his wife, and they will become one flesh." Separation from parents causes reliance upon God's sufficiency and creates a maturing union similar to our personal relationship with God the Father. Genesis 2:24 (NIV)

The husband is given "headship" over the family just as Christ is head of the church. He has been given spiritual responsibility for the family and must provide for their needs even to the point of self-sacrifice (Ephesians 5:25). This is not a means of pulling rank but a cascade of teaching love, forgiveness and self-sacrifice from Christ through the father and the mother to the children.

Tradition and Scripture hold the role for the wife-mother to be the person who bears and nurtures the children, keeps the home and takes care of the day to day needs of her family.

"A wise woman builds her house, but with her own hands the foolish one tears hers down." Proverbs 14:1 (NIV)

"She watches over the affairs of the household and does not eat the bread of idleness. Her children arise and call her blessed; her husband also, and he praises her ..." Proverbs 31:27, 28 (NIV)

Though the wife is to take chief responsibility with the caretaking tasks of home, this does not exclude the husband or children from helping around the house nor exclude the wife from some economic activity outside the house.

The roles of the husband and wife differ in accordance with the specific abilities given to them by their Creator. Children observe these roles and the differences in abilities, physical attributes and emotional expressions. They watch attentively because they are seeking to understand the differences in the sexes they can personally identify with.

GENDER IMITATION

For a seven-year-old, Sherry was a very bright and pleasant little girl. But she was a typical second grader when it came to household responsibilities, sometimes forgetting even after her mother had asked, warned, and scolded.

One day, Sherry's mother noticed she didn't have to ask

her daughter to help. The table was set without asking, her homework done, her room kept neat, and she even offered to feed the cat.

After about a week of this greatly improved behavior, Sherry's mom asked her about it.

"I saw Daddy hug you and say how much he loved you for all your hard work."

It's often the little things you do that mean the most and teach the best lessons to your children. Sherry saw the reward her mother received from doing "housework." Then she decided to imitate her mother, hoping to receive the same affectionate reward. Sherry may not be ecstatic about working around the house, but her attitude toward "womanly duties" is likely to be positive.

Once pre-school children learn which qualities define male or female roles, they often imitate these behaviors, looking to see what kind of response they'll get from parents, siblings and friends. Positive responses for wearing "army" clothing will help a young boy decide how to dress. Negative responses from other male friends for playing with dolls usually stops it cold. The imitation and testing of various adult-like behaviors is an innate part of maturing socially.

How can parents help their pre-school children to imitate these gender qualities that are pleasing to God?

Parents can encourage them and suggest activities to help them know what men and women do. I often encourage my girls to help their mother when she bakes, especially when she makes cookies. Don't discourage your children from trying any activity usually done by the opposite sex. As you point out which jobs or activities they can do, mention which sex usually does that job. This will help to define sexually related abilities, interests and careers.

I remember bragging on my older daughter to some friends one evening, stating "Bethany is so smart. She is going to be a doctor some day." I wasn't expecting the reply.

"Daddy, I want to be a nurse so that I can really help people. Besides, girls grow up to be nurses."

So after getting over the shock of realizing I didn't really help people, I had a chance to tell her that some of the best doctors I know are women doctors.

Your children will bring home various ideas of who should do what, regarding proper and improper roles for men and women. Be ready to support what is scriptural and to correct what is wrong.

Use Bible stories and the description of Bible characters as a "gold standard" for teaching gender roles to children. The masculine character qualities exemplified in the lives of Adam, Noah, Abraham, Moses, King David, the Lord Jesus and others give parents numerous examples of male gender behavior from which children can learn.

Female characters, such as Eve, Sarah, Esther, Ruth, Mary, and others, display many character qualities of the "virtuous woman" as described in Proverbs 31.

There is a double blessing in using these characters for examples. Children will not only see the gender characteristics for men and women, but they will also see the spiritual qualities and responsibilities that differ between men and women.

CURIOSITY

Parents often become worried when their pre-school child shows a preoccupation with "going to the bathroom" or with private body parts. Young children are learning to interact with their environment. They are beginning to understand themselves and they are curious about all things. This curiosity leads them to expose and play with their private parts and to share this new "knowledge" with other playmates. Comparison between pre-schoolers of the opposite sex is not an uncommon occurrence. Parents may believe in error that their child is sexually maladjusted.

Curosity of this sort is common and healthy to a point. The normal learning process includes learning about the body and its functions, yet parents should use discovery of self-exposure as a means of teaching children the inappropriateness of undressing in front of the other sex. It can also be an opportunity to explain that physical differences exist between boys and girls.

Repeated purposeful exposure of the private areas may develop into a form of disobedience. Deal with it as a disobedient act and give adequate discipline.

LOVE

It is not difficult for children to see love from a parent, but it is extremely difficult for pre-school children to verbalize an understanding of this abstract concept. Yet love is the very foundation of understanding the family, marriage, sexual union, self-sacrifice and salvation. Love must be present for a child to grow, learn, mature, and accept Christ. Our example of love teaches our children how to receive the love of Christ.

Teaching children how to be loved, to love God, to love others and to love self is probably the most important task that God has given to parents. Love must be differentiated from lust — desire for intimate affection and sexual contact. Pre-schoolers will understand physical love via affection, hugs, kisses, squeezing, holding, etc. Physical affection is important and must be fulfilled by parents or the child will suffer from emotional deprivation.

To a child, love is something that is received: a kiss, a hug, a present. God's concept of love is giving, not receiving. The world wants love to be self-fulfilling. Christ commands that love be self-sacrificing. It is essential that we teach our children both wings of love, so that they may receive the love of God through Christ and yet reach out to those in need with self-sacrifical love.

Love can be compared to giving, sharing and acting kindly to a friend or sibling. Teaching children to give a sick child one of their toys, to share toys with a brother or sister, are concrete demonstrations of the presence of love.

Comparing quantities and qualities of love helps children to solidify the concept in their minds. A physical example of giving love might be a brother who gives a bite of ice cream to the child, compared to a parent who would give a dish of ice cream to the child, compared to the Heavenly Father who could give all the ice cream in the world to the child.

The greatest act of love shown to man, the sacrificial death of the Lord Jesus Christ on the cross, is the best example of giving love we can teach our children. The spiritual definition of love always contains references to giving (John 3:16). All the examples of love that we show to our children and any personal examples of love between parents should highlight the "giving" aspect of love.

EARLY-SCHOOL LEVEL AGES 7 TO 10

Children in this age group are expanding their ideas and knowledge at a staggering rate. Within the last year, our older daughter has gone from the beginning of her addition tables to well into her multiplication tables, from reading,"Run, Jack, run," to a fourth-grade edition of *Robin Hood* . Playing soccer, piano, gymnastics and giving a full recital on her violin were among her other activities within the last year. Though she is shy about praying, her spoken prayers show a good understanding of missionary needs, both physical and spiritual needs. All of this has occurred in one year.

Experts in child development have classified the early-school level as the "socialization period," where children learn the intellectual and cultural skills that are necessary for them to function as adults. Most modern societies utilize these years of rapid skill development to teach children specific intellectual skills — reading, writing, mathematics — as well as creative skills such as art, athletics, hobbies and home skills. It is also a time for attaining social skills and learning to interact within a society through the family and through peer-group relationships.

Children's sexual attitudes continue to mature during this period of development as they socialize and exchange their ideas with others. Their gender identity continues to develop as they observe their parents, peers and peers' families.

Young children test their new relationships during this time as they are exposed to a widening circle of friends. As they interact with members of the opposite sex, they may go through their first emotional relationship, or first "crush."

Morality, the ability to choose right over wrong, begins to be developed as these children are making more of their own decisions. Building a sense of morality is a complex interweaving of family, societal, religious and peer-group values into a system of "personal values" that affects behavior, communication and relationships.

There is no more golden time to teach our children the scriptural values for sexuality, morality and all the areas of Christian living. We will forfeit our best opportunity to the schools or to the peers of our children if we wait until early adolescence.

PEER-GROUP INTERACTION

I am sure you have heard some of the same things that I hear from our children. The jokes they learn in school, the stories they have been reading, the personal and family problems of their classmates are all entered into their susceptible memories. How much richer their minds are for these interactions, but how much more we have to worry about the wrong ideas, the anti-biblical philosophies that could creep in and cause confusion and a likelihood for sin. There is no more worrisome area for parents than their children's sexual attitudes.

Peer-group interaction plays a large role in developing the sexual attitudes of children. School and play times give them an arena in which to test and refine these ideas. A male child who copies in play the "macho" image of a cartoon character on television is likely to be rewarded with loud cheers from his friends who will then themselves begin to copy what he does. Female children dress up and model the feminine characters they see in advertisements or on TV. As their friends admire them, they will copy those "female" traits. Few rewards for behavior are greater or more compelling than the positive comments of friends within the group. Comments such as "neat, cool, bad, out-of-sight, etc.," reinforce these sexual behaviors.

As parents, we need to keep a close watch on these powerful mind-shaping reinforcements given our children by their friends. By allowing children to play with friends that will support scriptural values and by watching their play we can stay in control of some of the sexual input of the ideas that will shape their attitudes.

Your male child is imitating "Skeleton-Man," an evil character that hates society, hurts people and loves money. As you observe your son destroy the "good guys," you can ask some questions about morality and gender characteristics: What is good and evil? Is Skeleton-Man good or evil? What bad things does he do? Do Christian men and women hurt other people? Are men always mean? Did the Lord Jesus act like Skeleton-Man? Wouldn't you like to play like the "good guys?" Does daddy act like the Lord Jesus or Skeleton-Man? How would Skelton-Woman be different from Skeleton-Man?

We can use many of these teachable moments to reinforce the biblical, moral characteristics that help our children understand their gender and mature in the understanding of the things of Christ.

FAMILY RELATIONSHIPS

Between the ages of seven and 10, parents begin to take their children to social functions, concerts, adult church, banquets and even to friends' homes. They are finally able to sit still and act maturely for at least a few hours. These added social experiences continue the maturing process by exposing children to adult situations and by allowing them to see and imitate these adult behaviors.

Plague in Our Midst

Looking and acting older is something children strive for within the family and peer-group. They begin to dress in clothing that stresses the physical differences between the sexes. Emotionally they attempt to imitate adults. They cry less often. They show more poise and composure. They demonstrate more respect for adults and more responsibility for their actions.

Sibling camaraderie is common. Brothers play basketball, build models, ride skateboards together. Sisters share clothing, listen to the same records, and occasionally talk about boys. A strong gender-peer-group starts with siblings in the same family and extends to neighborhood and school friends.

The examples that we show our children become extremely important in this group, as children, pushed by their peers to act more maturely, must rely on the example of their parents to show them how to be more mature. The relationship of mother and father — loving, sharing, communicating qualities of a stable marriage — are seen by children, processed and then stored for future imitation.

Children from seven to 10 are very open to examples of behavior they observe in other spheres — in older kids at school, television programing, characters, advertisements and music. These "worldly" influences are seen as keys to peer group acceptance. Imitation of these behaviors is "in." Even our Christian children are drawn to "act-out" the same outrageous hair-styles, clothing, language or behaviors simply to gain acceptance from their friends.

The 10-year-old son of friends of ours came home with his hair in long, purple spikes. His mother just started to cry. "Don't we love you enough? You had to do this to yourself just to get your friends' approval? We love you just the way you are."

That quickly cured the purple-spike syndrome.

We need to teach our children that approval is never to be based on outrageous dress or on groupie behaviors such as drug use or sex. It may cost them something to give up this type of behavior. Probably it will hurt their chances for acceptance by being obedient to their parents and to God. By doing what is right, they will have an excellent opportunity to show everyone that they are mature.

Showing God's unconditional love to our children when they do come home with purple spikes builds a trusting, communicating relationship and allows them to mature, putting away childish rebellion. It usually cures the spikes as well.

INTELLECTUAL DEVELOPMENT

My wife and I have decided to educate our children through a local, Christian day-school. Our decision was made because an excellent school was nearby and because the public school text-books present such anti-scriptural values in just about every subject area.

Humanistic educators, those who control textbook content, have used these books to destroy the traditional, biblical and family values that have been taught since the inception of public schools. This sad fact has caused many concerned parents to flee from "free" education because the cost is too high.

Parents need to be aware of the content of textbooks in both public as well as Christian schools. They often depict single-parent families or homosexual relationships as a norm in society. This is not appropriate. Displays and discussions of promiscuous sexuality can also be found. Though we want to foster our children's intellectual development, we must take care to ensure that proper scriptural values are taught through course work and textbooks.

MALE-FEMALE RELATIONSHIPS

Emotional and sexual desires begin to influence seven- to 10-year-old children, and the many cries of "Girls? Oh yeuch!" turn into "Who is it this week?" Many of these puppy-love relationships mark the first daring venture of young boys and girls into experimentation with "adult male-female relationships." Often these relationships represent the desire of a child to "play house" in imitation of adult behaviors.

The driving force for finding a boyfriend/girlfriend becomes the acceptance offered within the peer group. Acceptance by members of the same sex is often dependent upon acceptance by the opposite sex. The peer group defines certain parameters of accepted behavior and almost universally proclaims "mature, adult-like actions" are the ticket for success. This pseudo-maturity is fulfilled by parroting adult actions, dress and relationships.

These early "puppy-love" relationships often are not sexually motivated and may be inspired by peer-group acceptance. Because a child lacks emotional maturity, we need to watch out for promiscuity. Children are not mature enough to make choices that have long-term consequences. Yet, some nine-to 12-year-olds begin to experiment with touching, caressing and other affectionate behaviors. I'm aware of a number of 10- and 11-year-old girls who had blossomed physically and were made pregnant by an older adolescent.

Health educators suggest that classroom discussions of intercourse in this age group are necessary to prevent the sexual mishaps of children having children. But logic and experience show us that it is a foolish and dangerous suggestion. The combination of curiosity and immaturity will stimulate children to try what they are emotionally unable to handle. They are intellectually unable to consider the consequences.

Teaching children in this age group about male-female relationships should focus on the ultimate relationship goal — that of marriage. General discussions of dating, building friendships with the opposite sex, and the characteristics of an ultimate mate will keep the child thinking toward a long-term relationship a long time in the future.

We can discuss their having affection for the opposite sex and rules forbidding certain types of affection. These discussions will be too late if they have been postponed until adolescence. But an open, "bare-all" discussion of affections leading to intercourse, along with frank information about sexual intimacy, is likely to stimulate children more than convince them to abstain. A balance between too much and too little must be maintained.

This age presents an excellent time for us to share the scriptural teachings about marriage, temptation and abstinence. Marriage can be seen as the ultimate, God-given goal for any relationship with sexual relations as a beautiful reward. The admonitions in Proverbs to resist temptation, and to remain abstinent can be discussed along with the many benefits shown in Scripture. Obedience and sacrificing short-term pleasure can be used as the simple, memorable concepts that will make decision-making easier for your young person.

DEVELOPMENT OF MORALITY

A teacher in a sex education class one afternoon turned the discussion to the definition of morality.

"Now what is the most moral choice? Should a woman choose to use birth control pills so that she will not conceive, should she have an abortion or should she have an unwanted child who will be beaten and probably forgotten?"

One of the students quietly raised her hand.

"Mr. Lawson? You forgot some of the choices. She could give her child up for adoption? I know a couple of families who would make that a wanted baby."

When the little girl got home that afternoon, she discussed the teacher's choices with her mother.

"Don't worry, sweetheart," her mother said. "The world doesn't think much of children. God gave His best, the Lord Jesus, for each child. He thinks children are worth everything."

Plague in Our Midst

"Maybe, if Mr. Lawson had to decide to abort his own child he would choose differently," the girl said.

Morality is the ability to make proper, God-honoring choices; and that ability must be cultivated. Scriptural principles are the most important factor, but often they are not the only factor that must be considered. Input from other areas of knowledge — social customs, scientific advances, legal constraints and personal preferences — may also influence moral choices.

The difficulty of making a moral decision is erased when Scripture is applied to a question or dilemma. Mr. Lawson's choices and ultimate decision were faulty because they were devoid of a biblical choice. The skillful application of scriptural wisdom to a problem is like the swift and decisive stroke of a diamond cutter's mallet that expertly creates a gem.

As we are assured that scriptural principles are moral, it becomes an easier exercise when we follow these truths to assure us of moral integrity.

Sexual decisions can also be moral when scriptural truth is applied. Obedience to God's word is the ultimate moral decision and it protects us from sexual sin and from other ills in relationships. Sacrificially keeping yourself pure is not only moral, but it is obedient and builds spiritual faith. Obedience, self-sacrifice and faith continue to grow in importance as sexual decisions become more difficult in adolescence.

CHAPTER SEVEN
Adolescent Sexual Attitudes

    Adolescence is probably the most difficult time in the life of any individual. The complex society we live in places extraordinary demands on the the psyche of adolescent "children" who are just beginning to turn into adults. Peer and social pressures to be liked, perform, be responsible, make adult decisions are often too much for these immature young persons. They need our nurturance, emotional support and repeated reminders of guiding values until they eventually leave the nest.

    Teaching adolescents about sexuality always fills the hearts of parents with fear and trepidation. But it doesn't need to. We can use our knowledge about these attitudes, sexual function and Scripture to build a bridge of communication and trust with our adolescent children. We don't need to preach to or talk to them like babies. We should encourage them to remember how to make God-honoring choices, through obedience, self-sacrifice and faith in hope that our encouragement and love will give them the strength they need to please God in their bodies.

ADOLESCENT LEVEL — AGES 11-17

I am always in awe to see the sun setting over the Blue Ridge Mountains on a warm, summer evening. Yet, within minutes, the beautiful colors may turn into drenching showers and clapping thunder, destroying the illusion of a peaceful evening.

The beauty of a maturation is predictably interrupted with the storms, trials and testing in the adolescent; storms may be the rule instead of the exception. Their changes in attitudes toward their family, peers, bodies, purpose, authorities create an unstable base from which to mature. Their lack of internal stability and constant grasping for self-esteem brings storm after storm, conflicts within and without until they ultimately emerge from the chrysalis as a mature and beautiful adult.

> "Consider it pure joy, my brothers, whenever you face trials of many kinds, because you know that the testing of your faith develops perseverance. Perseverance must finish its work so that you may be mature and complete, not lacking anything." James 1:2-4 (NIV)

One of God's most difficult principles for each of us to learn is we cannot mature in faith unless we suffer through conflict. Each of us, in the adolescence of our spiritual growth, has been tempted, tossed, and trampled for the sake of growth in Christ. And haven't we rebelled against God's compassionate hand that was, for our own perfection, leading us through these different trials?

But God's purpose is fulfilled through these conflicts of adolescence. Each of us completes an essential period of physical, emotional, and spiritual maturation that opens the door to adult responsibility. As well, each person must mature in his sexual attitudes through this period. The same stormy course of conflict begetting maturation occurs

Plague in Our Midst

in our sexual attitudes and provides the foundation for our sexual conduct as adults. It is our choice whether these principles will be scripturally based promoting self-protection, obedience and faith or will be devoid of values leading to sex by the "world's" rules.

ATTITUDES TOWARD PHYSICAL MATURATION

There is nothing quite as earth shaking as observing your body change before your eyes, especially when it becomes different, awkward and even ugly. These changes spark many emotional questions, such as, "What will I become?" "Why is this happening?" "Will I be acceptable to my friends?" "Why do I feel so strangely?"

Many of us can remember our own personal turmoils. Even one "zit" was too many — but a whole face full? Your hair was never right. You were always too heavy. And you were scared to death to ask that cute girl in your algebra class for a date. How about all those episodes of "real love," those strong physical desires to hold and to be held.

Parents can prepare a young person for transition through this physically awkward stage by teaching adolescents about God's plan for maturity — that growth through various testings and trials is a normal and scriptural process resulting in maturity. We must teach them about the normal body changes, the purpose of the changes and the order in which the changes will occur. Early adolescence is an important time to begin discussing trials, temptations and bodily changes; but, as suggested in the last chapter, it is not the right time to tempt them with descriptions of intercourse.

If the parents default and allow the child's concept of adolescence to be shaped by the "world," then the "use it while you have it" mentality and peer pressures will tempt the young adult into sinful choices.

In the next chapter, there is specific information about

physical maturation and how parents can discuss this topic with their teen.

Physical maturation occurs long before emotional-social maturation is completed. Physical maturation occurs between the ages of 12 and 15 for young women and 13 and 17 for young men. Almost all young adults at this stage are emotionally unable to handle marriage or work in our complex society.

Yet, the ability to conceive and become pregnant occurs years before a young adult is emotionally mature and socially responsibile in our society. I have never seen a 13- or 14-year-old who is emotionally and financially able to handle separation from parents. But, I deal with scores of these children who are sexually active. This is one reason why divorce is so common when young adults marry.

We need to teach our children this important concept and help them to postpone sexual activity until marriage when they can handle all the necessary responsibilities.

ATTITUDES AND EMOTIONAL CHANGES

Dealing with adolescent family problems in the office is one of the most difficult and demanding of all the counseling situations that I deal with. Parents that I counsel are often distraught. They shake their heads stating, "His behavior just doesn't make sense."

Adolescent behavior doesn't make sense. It is usually inconsistent. Adolescents act on feelings, urges and desires, peer suggestions, often contrary to parental suggestions, just to "be unique."

Searching for a unique, personal identity is the adolescent's primary task of emotional maturity as he tries to grow up. As he begins to test new ideas, often different from the parental values, he brings conflict into the family. Communication breaks down. Parental authority is weakened, widening the understanding gap. Pulled by his peers to rebel, to act out, and otherwise go against established

Plague in Our Midst

principles tempts the adolescent into rash behavior. And if these did not generate enough emotional confusion, new sexual urges and the need for opposite-sex companionship push more fuel under the flame of the young adult's sin nature.

The eventual reward of this arduous task is the creation of a new adult who has the self-assurance and motivation to launch away from family into a competitive world. But woe to the person who dares get in the way of this ever-advancing wave of change.

Inevitably, parents get caught in the middle of this fearsome wave. Out of love they bear the brunt of rebellious behavior. We are called to encourage our kids through the emotional ups-and-downs and consistently reiterate the principles of obedience, self-sacrifice and faith through example and discussions. As loving parents we should be there, no matter what decisions are made.

Does your adolescent follow the scriptural principles you offer regarding abstinence from heavy affection and intercourse or does he impress his peers by sneaking off to a forbidden party to "make-out" with a steady girlfriend?

Does your young adult damage his spiritual testimony by attending a drinking party with fellow athletes or does he follow your scriptural admonition "to flee from sin" by not getting into a compromising situation?

Does your adolescent hide the fact that she had accidental intercourse because she fears your harsh response? How can we protect our adolescents from their lusts, their irrationality, their emotional decisions? How can we teach them to protect themselves from promiscuity? How do we teach them to make scriptural decisions to abstain from sex?

SEXUAL VALUES FOR ADOLESCENTS

Rebecca had dated Sal for about three months. She knew they would eventually get married after high school, but she had never discussed marriage with Sal.

When they were parking one night, Sal pulled a condom out of his pocket and suggested they should have intercourse.

"I'm not ready yet," Rebecca said. Sal was embarrassed and promptly drove her home.

Should I do it now or should I wait until after he pops the question? Rebecca thinks. I love him, and I want to share with him; but I know I should wait. The more she tries to reason with herself, the more confused she becomes.

Rebecca is being stretched between her thin foundation of values and her thick overlay of emotional temptations. She's a typical teen female, where 50 percent don't succumb, and the other 50 percent do.

One of the best ways for parents to approach this problem with their teen is to teach proper, scripturally based decision-making. The need to abstain from sex is more serious today than 10 years ago, and it will be even more important in the future as AIDS continues to spread. Proper sexual decisions may save your young adult's life.

Those who are familiar with the logical process of making decisions, weighing both positive and negative outcomes of a situation, are more likely to make "right" decisions and to protect themselves from trouble.

Teaching our adolescents about abstinence, avoiding sexual intercourse, and shunning situations that could lead to sexual intercourse is the biblical and proper method of sexual self-control. Abstinence is the only, 100-percent proven way to protect oneself from pregnancy, venereal diseases and AIDS.

How does abstinence rate in the decision process? When weighing the decision to be and remain abstinent, we have to compare all the potential outcomes. By having sex, by giving up abstinence, our teens risk pregnancy, venereal diseases, permanent infertility, loss of future marriage partners, loss of self-esteem, guilt, emotional pain and possibly death by AIDS. The rewards for remaining abstinent are protection from diseases, pregnancy, death, guiltlessness, the potential of finding a better mate and respect of parents and others.

Spiritually, abstinence supports being obedient to God's word, sacrificing self-indulgence for a future partner and building faith through waiting for God's blessings.

Seldom, however, is a decision so simple and emotionally unencumbered. In reality, the decision is often between a strong, emotional, irrational desire to have sex and the values and reasons to abstain. Making the process simple, filling the mind with all the positive reasons to abstain, will give our young adult as much strength as possible to make the right decision.

Another way to simplify this process is by using the three principles — obedience, self-sacrifice and faith — as part of the decision-making process.

When you are offered a sexual relationship, ask yourself these three questions: Am I being obedient to my parents and to God by my decision? Am I sacrificing for my future mate as I hope he is sacrificing for me? Am I building my relationship with God by exercising my faith, by patiently waiting for God's reward? Am I being obedient, sacrificial and faithful by my choice?

The use of this spiritual "carrot" to remain abstinent can only help the young adult to choose correctly. Yet the major enemy in this battle remains the strong, almost uncontrollable feelings to have sex. Knowing that the feeling is there and knowing how it can tempt a person, can be extremely helpful in denying it the opportunity to bear fruit.

HORMONES AND LUST

One of the most distressing and exciting changes young adults face is the emotional-physical attraction they feel for the opposite sex. In a world that encourages young people to "follow your feelings," many succumb to the temptation to "do what comes naturally." Their feelings control their decisions.

Hormonal changes, as will be described in detail in the next chapter, create a sexual desire that cannot be dissected or studied. Different individuals have varying levels of sex drive, some none at all; and others have an almost insatiable desire for sex. The sex drive, however, obeys the laws of all our natural appetites. The more you starve sexual desire, the less you need to satisfy it; the more you feed it, the more gluttonous it becomes. So even these differences in sexual desire can be modulated by discipline.

Lust is the desire for a sexual relationship without building an emotional relationship first. Lust is a result of the hormone structure and the desire to fulfill that sexual appetite. Fulfilling sexual sin completes the cycle of lust. Desire has become sin.

Though the desire or temptation to look "lustfully" at a member of the opposite sex is due to our natural sex drive, the dwelling upon that desire becomes the sin, as would the act itself. It is here that we can build a defense.

Temptations will come. They should be expected. As these lustful feelings, sexual images and desires begin to well up, fleeing from them will cause them to cease and protect you from sin. There is no sin in being tempted, only dwelling on the temptation so that it could bear sinful fruit. We do not need to feel guilt when temptation arises, as long as it is promptly disposed of.

"...but each one is tempted when, by his own evil desire, he is dragged away and enticed. Then, after desire has conceived, it gives birth to sin; and sin, when it is full-grown, gives birth to death." James 1:14,15 (NIV)

Knowing that temptation is inevitable, we must learn to flee from it and put it out of our minds by thinking on other, non-tempting thoughts. God will not allow temptations that you are unable to put out of your mind. He has promised you that. Simply filling your mind with other things, reading Scripture, turning on the radio, having fun with a hobby, all are practical ways to kill a lustful desire.

Lust is the opposite of love, even though the "world" believes the two are identical. Lust is the selfish desire to fulfill a sinful act. Love is the unselfish giving of oneself for the good of the other. When love takes on sexual connotations, it can become lust. Worldly "love" loses its scriptural basis and turns into a self-gratifying emotion, ready to take instead of give. Self-sacrifice is love in the truest sense of the word.

PARENTAL AVAILABILITY

As an adult, it is easy to put away many of life's temptations by staying away from bars, turning off the television and not going to R- or X-rated movies. But, remember when you were in high school all the bad situations — the drinking, the sexual displays, the parties, the pornography — you "backed into."

If adolescents can learn to flee from the mental temptations that will occur, they still may need our help to flee from a situation where they could be trapped into succumbing.

After the basketball game, Brian caught a ride to a party with some of his friends. When they entered the supposedly chaperoned home, Brian saw a number of the players drinking beer. The chaperoning parents were quietly in a downstairs bedroom, watching TV and drinking as well. Some of Brian's friends went to the upstairs bedrooms with their girlfriends. Without a ride, someone to chaperone the risky and illegal behavior of many of his friends, Brian felt trapped.

His parents had discussed what should happen if he became stranded in a situation where he should not stay. He was quickly picked up by his parents after he called them. Brian knew when to leave and where to call.

Becky and her boyfriend had been dating for about four months. They had attended dances and sports matches but had never been alone without other friends or adults. After dinner, they had planned to go to a movie and then be home 30 minutes after the movie ended. Somehow, they ended up on a quiet side street and before long were "making out." Within a few minutes, Becky's boyfriend become more aggressive and started to take off some of her clothing. He seemed to have little self-control.

Becky's parent's had discussed the progression from kissing, to caressing, to undressing, to intercourse; and she knew that the worst could happen if she didn't stop right then.

After straightening herself, she stepped outside the car until her boyfriend promised to take her home. Her parents had also instructed her to get out of the car, walk to a nearby house, if necessary, and to call for a ride.

Even though he was temporarily embarrassed about his behavior, Becky's boyfriend never lost control again and became a complete gentleman on other dates. He had learned his lesson.

Let your children know that you are always available to pick them up if a bad situation should arise. There is no shame in making a mistake or in getting into a bad situation. Problems arise when one mistake compounds into other drug-related or sexual mistakes. Being supportive of their wise decision to call you will make it easier to call again if there is need. Parents helping their children to flee temptation has saved more than a few sexual, alcoholic, and drug-related mistakes.

SEXUAL PROBLEMS IN THE ADOLESCENT

Just as health educators and physicians are realizing that prevention can save millions of dollars through education so, too, parents can save untold guilt and emotional distress when they educate their teens to make "healthy" decisions. Decisions based on weighing positive and negative outcomes, not based in emotions, can help to prevent temptation from bearing sinful fruit. This approach can be used for many of the sexual problems that adolescents often "stumble" into.

DATING

A recent study showed that 70 percent of all young women who started dating at age 13 had engaged in sexual intercourse by the time they were 20. On the other hand, only 30 percent of those who began dating at or after age 16 had engaged in sexual relations.

When young people are alone they are tempted to sin. Here are some practical suggestions to help them "flee" temptation.

Opening your home to get to know your teen's date is always a safe way for them to begin a relationship. Taking time to accompany the young couple, while still giving them some alone time, is an excellent way to be supportive. The young adult knows that you are not far away, and trouble is unlikely to brew. Checking on a party or date at another home should be a routine, to make sure there are no suprises or unintended lies. Time limits are good and using them will make the young couple more accountable.

What is the appropriate age for single dating? Is the teen emotionally and spiritually mature? Is the place or situation where they will be dating safe? Is the date trustworthy? Are they old enough to date responsibly? Sixteen years may be too young for some but just right for others.

MASTURBATION

Adolescents often experience very powerful sexual urges to release sexual tension with self-stimulation (masturbation). Studies have suggested as many as 90 percent of all teen males have masturbated, and between 30-50 percent of all teen women. Many a disturbed parent has sought counsel for the child caught masturbating believing it due to some psychiatric problem.

Masturbation may start in children who show normal curiosity about their bodies and functions. Others learn about it through peer-circles and find it a way to release sexual tension.

Blindness, homosexuality, and various diseases are not results of masturbation. Guilt, premature ejaculation, sexual dysfunction and marital discord are possible complications of a long-standing habit of self-stimulation. From a spiritual standpoint, the imagination and visualization of sexual experiences often plays a role in masturbation; this fills the mind with obviously sinful and lust-building desire.

Prevention is still the best treatment. Educating young adults not to start is the best method of prevention. If a parent accidentally witnesses the act, he may make a firm suggestion to discontinue, before the child is addicted. If the habit is long-standing, then helping the adolescent deal with it can be attempted in a positive, supportive manner. Stopping an ingrained habit is best accomplished with goal setting, striving for less and less of the behavior until the need no longer exists. Going "cold turkey" with any addictive habit has worked for a few, but has disheartened the many.

PORNOGRAPHY

The availability of erotic magazines for children and young adults is a great problem in our society. Twenty years ago, pornography was relatively mild. Today's violent, total exposure pornography that promotes bizarre forms of sexuality and even exploits children for erotic purposes, gives great sexual excitement and is highly addictive. Few industries have changed the sexual mindset of our culture as completely as the pornography industry.

Our children need to know pornography is out there, that it portrays abnormal sexual behavior and can become addictive by feeding the lust, thereby desiring more and more. Protecting yourself from exposure, and never starting to view it is the best prevention. Be careful to never let it creep into your home in the form of stimulating ads or "swim suit" issues. My favorite health magazine just arrived and I was dismayed to see an entire section promoting new swimwear worn by female models in very provocative postures.

It's everywhere you look.

PREMARITAL LEVEL — AGES 18-22

There is probably no greater satifisfaction for Christian parents than seeing our children receive salvation and then launching into the world a mature, trustworthy adult. What a joy to see the fruits of the many years of emotional, physical and spiritual investment culminating in an adult who is able and willing to use the principles entrusted to him. What a blessing when they serve our Lord through their jobs, ministries and lives.

Physical maturation, the ability to bear children, is completed, yet emotional and vocational maturation may still be far from complete in an 18-year-old. Emotional maturity as suggested by mental health experts is the ability to form stable relationships, meeting each other's needs, giving, and sharing. Spiritual maturity is seen when Christ-likeness and self-sacrificial giving predominates.

Maturing young adults naturally seek to find a companion of the opposite sex with whom to share activities, occupations, interests, and especially love and affection. But, few parents seem prepared to guide their children in what to look for in a potential spouse. Qualities such as like-faith, good job, and lots of money are all that are mentioned. Many young adults are confused by the "world's" system of finding a partner based solely on mutual physical attraction or sexual compatability. We need to put "mate hunting" into proper spiritual perspective.

Once that perfect mate is found, the wedding planned and just around the corner, how can parents help almost-newlyweds put aside anxiety about marriage, living together and sexuality within marriage?Parents can play a great role in smoothing the transition from one family unit to another newly constructed unit by gentle give-and-take discussions of communication, spiritual oneness and sexuality.

SEARCHING FOR GOD'S PERFECT MATE

Have you ever noticed how absorbed young adults become in finding that "perfect" God-ordained mate? Their attention is almost completely distracted; their day-dreaming filled with thoughts of their dream-mate. It is a completely natural desire for companionship, love, affection and as Paul suggested:

> "Now to the unmarried and the widows I say: It is good for them to stay unmarried, as I am. But if they cannot control themselves, they should marry, for it is better to marry than to burn with passion." I Corinthians 7:8,9 (NIV)

The "world" is the first to offer its set of values for finding a worthwhile mate:
- "You must have a strong, insatiable desire to share yourself sexually with that potential mate."
- "Premarital sex is necessary to make sure there is sexual compatability."
- "It is helpful to have some common interests, compatible ideas about home life, children,. and to have compatible personalities."
- "These qualities are helpful but not essential as sexual compatability supposedly covers a multitude of other problems. Anyway, if love leaves, or sex becomes boring, you can always divorce and find another, more stimulating live-in, or spouse."

Many young Christian couples have based their choice of mates upon these obviously flawed worldly mandates and they develop marital problems when superficial difficulties rise to the surface. This could have been avoided if a parent had at least broached some of the spiritually appropriate qualities his child should seek in a potential mate. Spiritual qualities, character qualities and physical qualities should be thought through before the emotional flood drowns all chances for objectivity.

QUALITIES TO BE DESIRED

What are the spiritual qualities to be desired? The potential mate must obviously be born again. At no time should a Christian consider an unsaved person for a mate, and have the marriage plagued with an "unequal spiritual yoke."

Jim had found the perfect girl, the one that plucked his heart strings in unison. It was a long wait, but well worth the patience. She was beautiful. She was finishing her master's degree in physics and had the same musical hobbies as Jim. She even attended a conservative church. But her one flaw was a fatal one. Darlene did not desire salvation.

Patiently, Jim waited for her. They dated and were the best of friends. Yet Jim put off all serious talk of marriage until Darlene would trust Jesus as her Savior. During a time of separation, when Darlene was seeking direction through prayer, she was deeply convicted by Jim's faith, love and patience and decided to trust in the Christ who died for her sins. Half an hour later, for no apparent reason, Jim called and was overjoyed with the good news.

Jim's patience had paid off, and the wedding bells were soon ringing. His obedience to Scripture ensured their long-term spiritual compatability.

What are the other areas of spiritual compatability?

Is the prospective spouse interested in spiritual growth, Bible study, prayer, church activities, and at about the same level of commitment as you? Does he or she expect to have their prayers answered? Is he or she actively involved in ministering to needs, such as witnessing?

Does the potential mate have a similar level of need for companionship? A wife who needs a husband around the house should seriously consider that before marrying an evangelist.

Does the potential mate have the same or similar desire for ministry? One who desires to be an "outback" missionary in some desolate area should consider carefully before marrying someone who has not already been called for the same ministry.

Character qualities are also important to consider when becoming acquainted with those of the opposite sex. Do you and the potential mate have similar or compatible personality characteristics? Two very ambitious people many not be able to marry successfully because their careers may take them away from each other, or from the family. Other areas of character compatibility are temperament, communication styles, intellect, interests, hobbies and recreational preferences.

Do you and your potential mate have similar or compatible emotional characteristics? Do you have similar reactions to emotional situations such as withdrawal, aggressiveness, peacemaking, "falling to pieces," etc.?

Some semblance of physical compatibility is important but it is the least of these three areas: Is there sexual attractiveness between the two persons? Is there ability to restrain from premature or overly aggressive sexual activity? Is the physical attraction too strong to discipline? Is there compatibility between other physical needs, such as amounts of sleep, differing eating and exercise habits, household temperature, etc.? Too many differences will be a constant source of friction, creating disunity if too many incompatabilities exist.

By studying marriages and marriage partners, one could conclude that personality differences are either an important prerequisite or married persons did not look for areas of compatibility other than oneness in the bedroom. The secular divorce rate has exceeded 50 percent in recent years. This has resulted partially from the lack of parental direction in the areas of mate selection and from the overemphasis on sexual compatibility as the reason for marriage.

Christian homes should be teaching a different set of characteristics and qualities that our children can identify in a possible spouse. We can instill a desire for Christian character qualities by promoting these traits above physical beauty and sexual attractiveness. The values of spiritual rebirth, desire for spiritual things, a quiet and loving attitude toward others, good study and prayer habits, emotional stability, a generous and merciful heart, a good attitude toward job and responsibilities, and a forgiving spirit should be desired.

Marriage built upon the frivilous, self-indulgent need for good sexual relations crumbles when problems arise. A union that is built first upon the love of Christ, a solid spiritual foundation, and a measure of personality, emotional, and physical compatibility can usually weather any storm that comes its way.

MYTHS ABOUT THE PERFECT MATE

A number of questionable concepts have been passed around the Christian community suggesting rules for finding the perfect spouse. Some of these appear to have scriptural intent, while others demonstrate no biblical foundation.

Is there only one, perfect mate that God has supplied to meet our individual needs? No specific direction is given in Scripture as to finding the perfect mate, although some direction is given for behavior after marriage. Hebrew marriages were arranged by the parents and included a betrothal period for the young man and woman to become well acquainted. There is no model either for a "marriage for love" or a self-selected mate in Old or New Testament writings. Once a spiritual commitment was made to be married, it was expected that a physical and emotional melting together would occur and that the two would love each other.

The only acceptable marriages in our culture begin and end with an emotional-physical desire between the two young adults, often called lust. Lust is the opposite of a true spiritual love. This is an obvious reason why most marriages are doomed when they are consummated.

Scripture requires a spiritual unity to exist prior to marriage. It states that both be born-again believers. Allowing the Holy Spirit to direct our decisions in all matters of living and following God's will in our lives can only bring blessing to our relationships. No command to wait for the "only allowable mate" provided by God has been written in Scripture.

Many young persons have a mental picture of the perfect spouse for them. Their wish-list of traits has been well organized and often is so extensive that no prospective partner gets close to fulfilling the qualities on that list. Yet through prayer, seeking God's direction and organized preparation, such as comparing character qualities and through disciplined, non-sexual relationships with the opposite sex, the young adult can trust God to direct him or her to a very suitable partner.

I have had a number of friends who have never married because their concept of the perfect spouse was unobtainable. One young lady has prayed about her mate-to-be and knows that he will be an evangelist who preaches and teaches from Scripture as well as "Moody." She knows he will want to settle down and spend the rest of his life raising four, perfect children with her. She has not yet married and has just passed the age of 30.

Some have not married because a "perfect" spouse has not shown up. Others experience extreme emotional turmoil because they believe there is only "one" available spouse through the Lord's perfect will and they may have missed that person. Young adults should be taught and will rejoice to know that there may be more than one suitable Christian mate available. There may even be a long waiting list of prospectives.

Must sexual compatability be established before marriage can take place? Most Christians see the "world's" push for sexual liberation in this particular myth, but it has become so widespread that 60-80 percent of our own children are believing this. Even among born-again adolescents, 60 percent or more have succumbed to sexual experimentation prior to marriage.

There are so many instances where Christian young people have believed this lie and have given themselves sexually to their prospective mate. A great majority of these

Plague in Our Midst

relationships were dealt a swift, decisive death-blow by this premature sexual activity.

Josh McDowell, the foremost Christian expert on teen sexuality, has stated, "There is no need to try out what God has given you. The plumbing always works!"

Sexual compatibility has been assured by God's design of the sexual organs and by His design for growth and nurturance in marriage. There is no need to (and God has specifically commanded that two individuals should not) fornicate or test each other sexually before marriage.

Is love the most important determinant in selecting a potential mate? Love is an emotional response to the presence or knowledge of another person. It is a complex response consisting of memories of hormonal and intellectual responses, and sensory cues such as beauty, scent, touch, voice, etc. But with all emotional responses there is a natural waxing and waning of the intensity of the feeling.

Bobby and Jennifer were committed to marry after he had finished medical school. Jennifer had just completed her master's in Christian education. They had known each other for years, had been friends, dated, split-up, dated minimally for the past year and then recently decided to marry. Their compatibility from the emotional, spiritual and personality standpoint were well established facts.

After being apart for two months with only a few phone calls, Bobby sought counsel from his pastor because he wasn't sure if he still loved Jennifer.

"Love is not a feeling alone. Love is a commitment to be faithful, trustworthy and to always be there for your spouse. Feelings wax and wane as the partners are together or separated. The feelings will return as you are able to spend more time with Jennifer," the pastor said.

Many a young adult has thought of stopping the marriage because the "love" appeared to be less intense than before. This decrease in the intensity of love is normal and to be expected both in the premarital period and during the marriage. Some who marry for love seek divorce when the emotional response and the parallel excitement of sex lose their intensity.

Commitment and further growth in the relationship will cause the intensity of the "love" response to return and, most likely, to become more and more enjoyable and intense.

SEXUAL RELATIONS WITHIN MARRIAGE

Oh, the joy of seeing the rebellion of adolescence fade into the budding friendship between parents and their adult child. A warmer, more amiable relationship gives parents an excellent opportunity to continue offering values, particularly marital values, and scriptural principles to their maturing young adult. It is also an excellent time to talk openly, friend to friend, about the specifics of sexual function and relations.

Precise knowledge about sexual function, purpose and working of organs and passages, hormonal changes and influences, functional cycles and processes, are helpful in furthering the understanding of having children and of practicing birth control. Knowledge of sexual function is obviously not essential to having normal sexual intercourse; for if it had, the human race would have floundered years ago.

The secular press has created scores of books on the "how to's" of sexual intercourse. Most fiction contains many verbally explicit bedroom scenes describing how to touch this, how to position that. Intercourse has been reduced to a recreation, a great feeling. If this doesn't give you intense pleasure, try another method instead.

Newlyweds do not need everyone's opinion on what are the best moves for sexual relations. Young adults who have been exposed to pornography, prior sexual relationships and peer group "big talk" carry into marriage an excessive load of expectations about sex. If their greatly inflated expectations are not met, then their worst fears of sexual inadequacy have been realized. Newlyweds need the freedom to discover how best to share intimately with their spouses.

Plague in Our Midst

They don't need to be shackled with the "world's sexual baggage."

Teresa had watched her mother writhe with pain, beaten by her alcoholic father on many occasions. She had been told by her mother that all men were beasts, sexual animals who could not be trusted. Her mother's continual put-down of men shaped Teresa's opinions.

But she could not understand why she desired male company. The desire was strong. Once married, the sexual relationship for her became more and more difficult. Months had passed and then two years between sexual relations. Teresa's husband started drinking heavily out of frustration. Only through the counsel of a local Christian physician did Teresa finally realize the psychological "burden" given her by her mother. Within six months, their sex life was improving, the alcohol abuse had stopped and Teresa finally became pregnant.

Can parents tell their children too much? Fears, biases, personal sexual problems can be extremely damaging to the psyche of a developing young adult and can impair future sexual performance. Telling them your past personal sexual encounters, mistakes or exploits is probably inappropriate:. It may be helpful if you can keep it in non-personal, general terms. Telling them specifics about sexual relations is also unwarranted. Let the new couple have the joy and excitement of personal discovery.

What should parents teach their children about sexual function? The next chapter is organized to give parents and their children some background in the anatomy and physiology, the structures and function of the reproductive system. There will be a description of the bodily changes of puberty, the structure and function of both the male and female reproductive systems, methods of blocking fertilization and answers to some questions that teens often ask their parents about function.

CHAPTER EIGHT
Sexual Maturation and Function

As soon as she got home from school, Marsha ran directly to her room, sobbing. It took over an hour for Marsha's mother to coax her 10-year-old daughter to talk about the problem.
"Why are you so upset?"
"In social studies we talked about careers. Everyone was saying they wanted a career in business, medicine, art, and some other things too. I said that I wanted to be a mother and have four children. The whole room broke out laughing. Bobby said, 'Only babies have babies.' Someone else said, 'You don't get paid for being a mother.'"
It took a while but, when Marsha finally stopped sobbing, she and her mother had a long talk about "worldly values."

You would expect the world's disdain for children to be rampant as it is in most of the media. But what especially concerns me is the spill-over of this philosophy into the hearts of many Christians.

I have heard comments like, "I won't have children because they are too demanding" or "I could never put that kind of burden on my husband or wife."

Others I have talked with want to keep their family sizes to two children at most, due primarily to monetary considerations. One comment I've heard from two different people shows how far this idea has incorporated in a believer's life: "I don't want to have any children because I am having too much fun without them and I don't want to spoil it."

But I've also seen these "self-centered" ideas of family completely melt away with the arrival of a newborn to these Christian families, no matter if the pregnancy was planned or accidental. The joy of children utterly overwhelms all desire for selfish pleasures.

The miracle of human reproduction and the joy brought to a family by a child have been corrupted by secular influences. Many adolescent children, pregnant for the second or third time, see this potential blessing as a burden to carry, as an unwanted child, a piece of worthless tissue to be extracted. Even stable families with two children have considered aborting their third child because of the financial inconvenience he or she would cause.

The materialistic philosophy that promotes career success as the ultimate goal has down-graded the raising of children from a privilege to a financial burden.

The problems created by promiscuous sexuality along with these humanistic changes in social philosophy have made it essential for Christians to be informed about sexuality. AIDS threatens to kill our own children with one sexual mistake or one shared needle from an infected intravenous drug user. One mistake and, in three to five years, death. This message needs to be plain, easy to understand and firm.

Knowledge about sexual function, the masterfully

designed hormonal cycles, the self-sufficiency of an ovum, the miracle of fertilization, the amazing process of maturation and growth, provide the basic material and understanding parents will need as they teach their children about sexual function.

I have presented this material in a progressive sequence, fertilization to maturation and have attempted to confine the information to the essentials. This will give you a brief background in sexual function that will assist you in discussions with your children. A short section on birth control is included to help you answer your children's questions.

FERTILIZATION TO BIRTH

From the moment of conception, the sex of the child has been determined by the specific sperm cell that has penetrated the ovum or egg. Each of these sex cells has only one half of the genetic material, or genes, needed to make a new person. Addition of the two halves makes one whole gene pool, consisting of a wondrous substance called DNA, the God-created computer that makes every substance in our body and allows it all to work together.

Sperm, the sex cells from the male, can contribute either an X chromosome or a Y chromosome. The ovum has only an X chromosome. A female child comes into existence if the male's X and the female's X chromosomes combine, an XX code that denotes the female sex chromosomes. A male child is created with an X from the mother and a Y from the father, an XY configuration of the male sex chromosome.

Once the sperm and the ovum join, a new baby boy or girl is begun and a long sequence of maturation and growth that takes 40 weeks commences. During this time, cells are dividing and changing into all the different types of cells that will become the growing baby. Skin, muscle, heart, liver blood and even sex cells — both the sperm and ovum of the next generation — and all the other cells of the reproductive organs. Unborn children already house the cells for their own children within their reproductive organs.

Certain mishaps, accidents or deformities can occur during the fertilization and maturation processes. A new child may be short-changed and get only one sex chromosome or an extra sex chromosome. This will produce a mature child with some characteristics of either a male or female, but one who will be unable to bear children in the future. Rarely a child is missing certain parts of their reproductive organs, such as ovaries, fallopian tubes, uterus, or testes. Without normal reproductive organs, intercourse, conception and pregnancy are difficult or impossible. Other deformities may occur in the exterior organs, or genitalia due to abnormal hormones or for other reasons. These can make it difficult to distinguish the true sex of the new child.

SEXUAL CHANGES DURING PUBERTY

The sexual organs, the female ovaries and the male testes, remain dormant during the childhood growing period because they lack stimulating hormones. Once the child enters puberty, the term used for the maturation of the sexual organs and hormone systems, a great many physical, emotional, and hormonal changes occur.

The reproductive system is regulated by the "master gland," the pituitary gland that is deep within the brain, very close to the sinuses. Regulation of all the sexual organs and many other hormones occurs with the release of regulating or trophic hormones from the pituitary at the proper time of life. These trophic hormones stimulate the maturation of the testes and ovaries.

The pituitary then regulates the testes and ovaries and they regulate the hormones. Testosterone, the male hormone, is responsible for maturation of the sperm; the enlargement of the male sexual organs including the penis; the secondary sexual characteristic such as facial and body hair, deep voice, large muscles; and for the "hormonal urge" or sex drive.

The ovaries are responsible for the secretion of two hormones, estrogen and progesterone. The estrogen is responsible for maturation of the ovum on a cyclic or monthly basis. Estrogen is also responsible for the secondary female characteristics, such as breast gland development, smooth skin, fat deposition in the hips, thighs and breasts. The rise and fall of estrogen and subsequent rise and fall of progesterone stimulate an ovum to mature and to be released on a monthly basis.

The changes that are obvious to maturing young adults are the changes in their bodies. Puberty begins between the ages of nine to 16 years of age and then proceeds through an orderly process. Some young men and women are almost completely mature sexually before others begin. This may lead to self-esteem problems, anti-social behavior and withdrawal on the part of the late bloomers.

Male puberty begins a year or two after the female counterpart. A steady growth in weight, muscle strength and height takes place. The voice goes through a rapid change as the voice box enlarges to create a deeper, more masculine voice. Facial, body and pubic hair become thicker and more plentious through puberty. The sexual organs — the testes housed in the scrotum and the penis — enlarge to adult size. Once started, the entire process of puberty is completed in two to four years with some late growth spurts still possible.

Males often find a small amount of tissue under the nipple, usually just one, that enlarges and grows tender during puberty. This benign process, called gynecomastia, will eventually subside in months to years and is normal during puberty. Large or growing masses should be checked by a physician.

The testes of the growing male are often of different size, creating some concern by the adolescent and his parents. This is also a normal pattern of growth and may permanently persist into adulthood. Any question about the size, another mass in the scrotum, or a bump on the testicle should be checked by a physician as a number of benign and potentially serious problems may be occurring.

Female changes in puberty are similar in time frame to the male changes, except they start earlier. Puberty is a time for rapid growth in height, weight and fat distribution in the female. The breasts, or mammary glands, bud and begin to grow, signaling the onset of puberty. The internal sexual organs, the ovaries, fallopian tubes, uterus, and vagina are all enlarging during this maturation phase. The external genitals enlarge slightly and pubic or genital hair grows. As the mammary glands are maturing, the body is distributing fat or adipose tissue to areas stimulated by the estrogen hormone. The breasts, thighs, hips, and lower abdomen or stomach all begin to change shape due to the new fatty deposits. These fatty stores are intended as nutritional reserves during pregnancy.

After some physical changes have occurred, the young woman will experience her first menstrual flow between one to three years following breast bud development. Initally these monthly cycles are erratic as ovulation, the process of ovum maturation and release, does not occur or is itself erratic. Ovulation may not occur on a regular monthly cycle for years after the onset of menstrual flow or period. The begining of menstrual flow is called menarche.

Young women may become concerned about breasts that are unequal or periods that are very irregular. Breasts may develop at different rates, and may be slightly different sizes when mature, just like the male testes. Very different breast sizes may indicate a problem that needs to be checked by a physician, but it can be surgically corrected if it continues into adulthood. The irregular periods after menarche are normal and, if they continue, may be due to irregular ovulation. If the period doesn't start for many years after breast bud development, a physician should make a thorough check to see if there is a more permanent or correctable problem. If a period has not occurred by the age of 18, an exam and testing would be recommended.

UNDERSTANDING MALE SEXUAL FUNCTION

The primary function for the sexual organs is the transfer of male sex cells, sperm, to the female. The sperm mature in the testes, the primary male sex organ. The testes are suspended within the thin-walled sac of the scrotum so that the temperature is a few degrees less than body temperature, which is 98.6 degrees. Sperm appear to need a lower temperature than body temperature to divide and mature optimally.

The sperm cell is a well-designed vehicle to carry the father's genes, the DNA, to the waiting ovum. The design consists of a head and a movable tail that pushes the sperm from the vagina through the uterus to a waiting ovum in the fallopian tubes. The head contains the genetic material and is covered by a sac of enzymes that dissolve the protective envelope around the ovum.

Sperm are very small compared to the female ovum and must be supplied by the millions to fertilize an egg. Low sperm counts make it difficult to impossible for fertilization to occur. Millions of sperm, releasing their acrosomal enzymes next to the ovum, make penetration by one sperm cell possible.

A long set of tubes and conduits is present to pipe the sperm to the female vagina during intercourse. The epididymis and vas deferens are the first storage areas and set of tubes taking the sperm from the testes to where the reproductive and urinary tracts join. Along the way, secretions are added to the maturing sperm from the seminal vesicles and prostate. The secreted fluid contains certain proteins that activate the sperm, fluid which allows the sperm to move, and fructose, a form of sugar, that provides energy for the tiny sperm tails. The fluid secretion that contains the sperm is called semen.

The male exterior organ, the penis, must become erect before penetration is possible. This hardening and enlarging with sexual and psychologic stimulation occurs when blood flows into the erectile compartments, but cannot flow out. During stimulation, the autonomic nervous system becomes involved, providing control of the blood flow in and out of the erectile tissue. At climax, a rush of adrenalin from the adrenal glands causes the "sexual rush" that produces the intense pleasure of intercourse.

The climax or orgasm stimulates muscles in the vas deferens, epididymis and urethra to contract in "waves," rhythmically expelling the semen into the vagina. Once orgasm is reached, there is no control over the expelling or ejaculation of sperm.

UNDERSTANDING FEMALE SEXUAL FUNCTION

The female reproductive system is much more complex than the male system because of the cyclic maturation of the ovum and its associated changes.

The ovum matures in the ovaries, the paired female sex organs that reside in the abdomen, and is released into the abdomen when fully mature. One follicle grows and releases a mature ovum approximately on the 14th day of each cycle, and each ovary usually contributes one ovum every other month. The hormones, estrogen and progesterone, are partially responsible for this ovum maturation, as well as two other trophic hormones called FSH and LH.

The usual course that the ovum follows, once it's released into the abdomen, includes capture by one of the fallopian tubes, the uterus, and then implantation into the uterine lining or endometrium if fertilized. The fallopian tubes sweep the ovum into a bell-like opening and tiny cilia or fingers gently push the egg down the tubes into the uterus over a period of one-to-two days. If the ovum remains unfertilized, there is no implantation; and the uterus sloughs its lining, causing a period or menstrual flow.

Hormonal changes during the cycle are the rule and the

Plague in Our Midst

up-and-down swings create a regular cycle of events related to preparation for pregnancy. A cycle lasts from 21 to more than 40 days, with 28 days being average. During the first part of the cycle, the estrogen begins to rise and peaks on day 12-13. Two other trophic or regulatory hormones follow this same pattern and, combined with the estrogen, promote maturation and release of one ovum on day 14 — or 14 days before the menstrual flow begins.

The lining of the uterus, called the endometrium, begins to thicken in preparation to receive a fertilized ovum during this 14-day phase. As soon as the two trophic hormones, LH and FSH, and estrogen levels fall, the other hormone progesterone begins to rise. This hormone helps to build and mature the lining of the uterus. A few days before the menstrual cycle starts, the progesterone level decreases dramatically, stimulating the sloughing off of the endometrium if a fertilized ovum is not present.

The endometrial lining of the uterus is designed to accept a fertilized ovum, allowing it to implant and derive nutrition from the mother. A non-fertilized ovum does not send any signals to the ovaries to keep the endometrium in place, whereas a fertilized ovum announces its presence and tells the ovaries to keep producing progesterone to preserve the endometrial lining for the duration of the pregnancy.

INTERCOURSE AND FERTILIZATION

The human sexual response combines emotional factors, psychological aspects and physical stimuli into a complex, automatic response that transfers male sperm to the female vagina. The physical changes associated with sexual arousal are controlled by both the central nervous system — our brain and thought patterns — and the autonomic nervous system — the nervous system that controls involuntary body changes such as heart rate, digestion and sexual response. The intermeshing of thoughts of love and pleasure with the physical sensations of sexual relations leads to a climax sensation called orgasm.

The male climax is essential for transfer of sperm to the female for possible fertilization. Prior to climax there is an increased release of adrenalin and an increase in the pleasurable emotional response to those hormones. At climax, even more adrenalin is released causing a "rush" of pleasure, a warm sensation and ejaculation. Rhythmical contractions of the epididymis, vas deferens, seminal vesicles and urethra expel semen into the vagina at ejaculation. Without orgasm, sperm are not transferred and fertilization cannot occur.

The female response to sexual intercourse causes a hormonal response identical to the male but does not cause any movement or transfer of ovum or sperm. At climax, rhythmical contractions occur in the vagina, uterus, and fallopian tubes.

Eggs in a rabbit are released with sexual stimulation; however, in the human the egg or ovum is released in the mid-point of the menstrual cycle, not in response to sexual relations. These contractions in the human female do not propel the sperm into the uterus or the fallopian tubes.

Adrenalin is the chief reason for sexual pleasure and is also the primary source of pleasure for many addictive "highs." These would include stimulant drugs, such as cocaine and amphetamines; running and strenuous exercise and other activities that are often considered normal and healthy, such as violence or horror entertainment, workaholism and extremes of stress; and other vicarious or personal sexual relations such as pornography and excessive sexual excitement. All of these potentially create some degree of psychological addiction to repeated use of the substance or activity because of the adrenalin high it creates.

Sexual intercourse must occur two days prior to ovulation, the release of the ovum, and up to one day after for any chance of fertilization to occur. The life span of sperm once ejaculation has placed them within the vagina is about two days. The ovum once ovulated degenerates if not stimulated by sperm within a 24-hour period.

Fertilization may, but does not always, occur if sperm are present along with the ovum in one of the fallopian tubes. The enzymes on the head of the sperm slowly dissolve the protective envelope surrounding the ovum until one out of three-million sperm can enter the egg. As soon as one sperm enters, the egg becomes hardened to penetration from other sperm. The two cells join their genetic materials, making one complete cell, and start growing and dividing, producing the many diverse cells of the new child.

The fertilized ovum travels down the fallopian tube and implants in the soft, fertile lining of the uterus, the endometrium. The developing embryo sets up shop, forming a protective sac and a placenta where nutrients and oxygen are transferred from the mother to the child. Here the child spends the next 40 weeks developing all the necessary organs and extremities, increasing in size until able to survive by itself outside of mother's protective internal environment.

GOD'S PERFECT DESIGN

It is a sorry situation when such a beautiful part of God's creation becomes abused, defiled and distorted when people waste on sinful self-indulgence what was intended for their edification. God's wonderful purposes for sexual relations should not be obscured in the mire of worldly self-gratification, but should be taught to children in the context of scriptural principles that honor our Creator.

Not discussing sexual function or shunning knowledge about God's creation does not help us or our children to understand God's plan for love, marriage and sex. It is our privilege to glorify God through understanding the magnitude of His creative skill in the design and function of the reproductive systems and the children they procreate.

"For you created my inmost being; you knit me together in my mother's womb. I praise you because I am fearfully

and wonderfully made; your works are wonderful, I know that full well. My frame was not hidden from you when I was made in the secret place. When I was woven together in the depths of the earth, your eyes saw my unformed body. All the days ordained for me were written in your book before one of them became to be." Psalm 139:13-16 (NIV)

BIRTH CONTROL

A broad selection of pharmacological agents, devices and methods for controlling fertilization have been developed over the past 30 years to give individuals control over the number and spacing of their children. Methods to block sperm travel or ovulation would accomplish the necessary objective of allowing intercourse, yet make fertilization highly improbable.

Some family planning professionals suggest abortion as a birth control method. This is obviously not a method of control but a direct assault on the reproductive system of the mother and the direct mutilation and destruction of an unborn child. Other drug methods are being developed that compel the uterus to expel the unborn child like its own endometrial lining, thus destroying the implanted human life. These are not birth control methods and should not be promoted in family planning clinics as "control" methods.

Most birth control methods do what they suggest. By blocking sperm or preventing ovulation they prevent fertilization and pregnancy. The following describes the general methods of blockage and the specifics of these methods.

BARRIER METHODS—SPERM BLOCKAGE

A number of birth control devices exist that block the sperm from entering the vagina or, once deposited, from proceeding up the female reproductive tract to the fallopian tubes.

Condoms are a safe and reasonably effective way of accomplishing birth control. The condom consists of a soft, thin latex or rubber form that fits over the penis during intercourse. The sperm are ejaculated but cannot get outside of the condom and are disposed of after intercourse. Condoms however, have been known to break; and the sexual act must be interrupted when the man puts on the condom prior to intercourse. Effectiveness is approximately 90 percent taking mishaps into account.

Do condoms protect people from AIDS? Numerous studies of condom leakage have shown that between 10 percent and 25 percent of all condoms break or significantly leak. The AIDS virus is carried in the semen which makes leaking condoms more like "Russian Roulette" than protection.

The diaphragm is a latex shield that is placed inside the vagina prior to intercourse and almost completely covers the opening to the uterus called the cervix. To ensure effectiveness, the diaphragm must be combined with a spermacidal jelly or foam. Diaphragms must be fitted by a physician making it a prescription item; but they, unlike condoms, are reusable. There appear to be fewer problems with breakage of the diaphragm compared to condoms, but the effectiveness, approximately 90 percent, is still similar. As the semen is still deposited in the vagina, diaphragms offer no protection from the AIDS virus.

Spermacidal jellies and foams can be used separately, killing most of the sperm in the vagina before they can travel to the uterus; use with another barrier agent is suggested for better results. No studies have been done to see if these medications also kill the AIDS virus along with the sperm.

A new product called the "sponge" has recently been introduced. A small sponge, shaped something like the diaphragm, is permeated with a spermicidal jelly and placed in the vagina prior to intercourse. The effectiveness is about the same as the other barrier methods. They offer no protection from the AIDS virus.

BIRTH CONTROL PILLS—OVULATION BLOCKAGE

The female ovulation-menstruation cycle is very sensitive to changes in hormonal concentrations at various points in the cycle. Birth control pills use this sensitivity to suppress ovulation and to prevent potential fertilization.

The present day birth control pill (BCP) contains synthetic estrogen and progesterone in steady dosages for 21 days or in varying dosages for 21 days. The dosages of estrogen when BCPs were first formulated was approximately 10 times the dosage used today. The side effects of these early pills are not seen in today's pills.

The BCP works by preventing ovulation, both maturation and release of the ovum. The steady dosage of both the estrogen and the progesterone prevents the rise of the trophic hormones and the estrogen necessary for the ovum to mature and release. If taken on a regular basis, every day, the pill is 99 percent effective, but it becomes less effective as pills are missed. Once three consecutive pills are missed, protection from fertilization is greatly diminished; and an alternative method, such as condoms, should be used for the rest of the month.

New studies show that there is no risk of breast, cervical or uterine cancer with the BCP's at these lower dosages. In fact, taking BCPs on a regular basis may confer some benefit in decreased risk for endometrial cancer and pelvic infections. These are early studies and more data needs to be collected and analyzed before this can be confirmed.

Though BCPs are the most effective form of birth control, they have two drawbacks — price and side effects. BCPs cost between $10 and $17 per month and the user must have a PAP/pelvic exam from her physician yearly rather than every three years (which is the present recommendation for non-users). The woman on the pill may have early side effects that pass with continued usage. These side effects can be headache, nausea, flushing, as well as persistent problems with headaches, weight gain, nausea, bloating, periods decreasing or stopping, and spotting or bleeding in the middle of the cycle (breakthrough bleeding).

Though birth control pills are the most effective non-abortive form of control, the "anti-child" philosphies of the world have helped to persuade the public to believe that birth control is safer and more natural than pregnancy. Birth control pill manufacturers circulate some very suspect data, supporting the "world's" notion that having children is a "pathological" condition or disease. Studies show that more women die from childbirth or its complications than die from taking the birth control pill or its complications. Careful scrutiny of the studies shows that the manufacturers break the pill-use group into smokers and non-smokers, thus halving the risk for each group and making pregnancy appear less safe. This attitude again shows the disdain for the unborn. It also gives the secular population one more reason not to have children and, of course, to buy more birth control pills.

For those who refuse to remain abstinent and continue to pursue promiscuous sexual activity, they will find no protection from the AIDS virus while using the birth control pill. Condoms alone remain the only way to prevent the spread of the AIDS virus from one person to another when having intercourse. Even then there is at least a 10 percent — and some say as much as 25 percent — failure rate in condoms.

ANTI-IMPLANTATION METHODS

Intrauterine devices (IUD) have been used by many women to prevent implantation if an ovum becomes fertilized. The IUD is a plastic and metal object that is placed inside the uterus. It irritates the lining of the uterus so that implantation cannot occur. The benefits of this type of birth control include its being put in place once by a physician and then left in place for three-to-five years. Forgetting to take pills or to insert the device ceases to be a problem.

There are a number of very serious side effects that potentially occur with the IUD, and many devices have been removed from the market for liability reasons. Once placed in the uterus, the IUD increases the chance for infection in the uterus and tubes. The IUD can perforate the uterus and, if fertilization occurs with implantation, the IUD can kill the unborn child (as can attempted removal of the IUD during pregnancy). Some women claim IUDs have caused permanent infertility. Others have them removed because of discomfort after insertion.

Philosophically and actually, the IUD can cause an abortion if fertilization has happened. Abortion cleans the womb of any tissue, especially the baby, by pulling it from the implantation site. An IUD does not allow the young child to implant in the endometrium. It pushes him or her through the uterus and destroys any chance for complete maturation.

Another type of hormonal birth control does something similar. Progesterone-only BCPs prevent implantation and the movement of the sperm up the female reproductive tract. Seldom does it suppress ovulation. When fertilization occurs, the new child is "mini-aborted" by not allowing implantation in the endometrium.

Pellets of injectible progesterone are becoming available as a long-term (five-year) birth control method. These pellets of hormone are injected under the skin and slowly release progesterone into the blood stream. The uterus under control of the synthetic hormone does not allow implantation of the fetus, thus aborting the baby.

PERMANENT STERILIZATION

The male and female both have paired conduit passages from the primary sex organs, the gonads, to the penis and uterus. These tubes, once cut and tied, can permanently block the passage of sperm or ovum.

Vasectomy is the name of the procedure for cutting the male vas deferens under local anesthesia.

There is little pain during or after the procedure and virtually no side effects from the permanent cutting. A few studies have shown an increased risk of heart disease following vasectomy, but more study into this question has disproved the possibility. Reversing the procedure is possible; but is difficult, expensive and it holds only a 25- to 50-percent chance of success.

Tubal ligation is the women's procedure for permanent sterilization. It can be accomplished through an incision or with a fiber-optic instrument called a laparoscope. Both destroy the tubes and, with the open incision, ties can be placed as well. The women must go through general or spinal anesthesia with more risk of complications than a local procedure such as vasectomy. There is more post-surgical pain with the tubal ligation. Women often suffer a short period of nausea with the open procedure and risk infection as well as long-term pain with scar tissue. Reversing tubal ligation is possible; but it is very difficult, expensive and holds little chance of success.

Hysterectomy or removal of the uterus can also be used as a means of permanent sterilization but it is usually reserved for the woman who has problems with her uterus or menstrual cycle. It is a much larger and more painful operation.

TIMING METHODS

A number of other "personal motivation," non-drug or device methods have been used without much success by couples who desire to postpone their family. Discipline is the key to success with all of these methods, especially for the male. Failure is common due to the strength of the male sex drive during sexual relations and the automatic, uncontrolled response of the climax.

Interrupting intercourse before the male ejaculates has been used for many years prior to the availabilitiy of birth control. Any spilling of semen within the vagina may leave enough sperm to cause a pregnancy. Other variations include allowing the male to reach climax, then squeezing the base of the penis to impede the semen flow. Extreme discipline is necessary and few are able to continually and effectively complete these methods to prevent pregnancy.

Probably the best of the timing methods is called the "calendar method." The ovum is usually released on the 14th day of a 28-day cycle; and as the ovum can be fertilized for one-to-two days, abstinence from intercourse must begin on day 11 to 12 and continuing through day 16 or 17. This method works poorly for women with an irregular cycle, men without discipline or couples who have very active sex lives. Couples who have infrequent intercourse, where the women has a regular cycle and where discipline is no problem, may be very successful with this non-device or non-drug method. The "calender method" costs nothing and is little bother. Those who practice this method cannot be assured of total birth control and should be willing to have a child if the possibility occurs.

NON-METHODS FOR BIRTH CONTROL

A few married couples practice a non-method relying totally upon faith in God.

These couples believe that He should regulate the number, spacing and timing of all children through totally natural methods.

Trust to meet all of their financial, housing, emotional, as well as the spiritual needs for the large families that result can be extremely rewarding for couples whose complete interest is in pleasing their Creator. I personally have great admiration for couples who practice this type of family planning for the witness and faith they radiate to the church.

Many Christian leaders are rediscovering this biblical concept of non-birth control and are speaking in support of this method in seminars, books and sermons promoting large families as one of God's designs for church growth. These speakers are careful to point out how the "world" has

Plague in Our Midst

tried to poison this scriptural ideal by suggesting birth control, two children per couple, population crises, zero growth, and many other materialistically oriented philosophies. It appears that since the world is trying so hard to prevent large families that the scriptural ideal for large families must be correct.

Initially, the large family was intended for protection from enemies, productivity in an agricultural society, social security in parental old age, and population insurance as many babies died during birth and infancy from disease. Our modern culture has very high birth rates, very low death rates for infants and children and a culture where children confer little protection in old age or from enemies.

But what better way exists for evangelizing the world than through large Christian families, where children who get a burden for a lost world can spread the gospel through home and foreign mission fields.

If there is one correct method for birth control for Christian couples, this non-method may be it. Those who practice it should not belittle those with lesser faith. They should not suggest to them that birth control is sinful but instead should help disciple that couple to grow in their faith.

For those couples who do choose a birth control method, I would like to offer one suggestion about witness. One woman told me that she used an IUD and did not want to know about how it worked, just as long as it did work.

But consider those who are weaker, less mature Christians or non-believers. These people do know that IUD, mini-pills and other methods are very similar to abortion. Even if this woman did not know, her witness to others was destroyed; and she may have led others into "abortion" without knowing it.

Information is important. How we live our lives, the major decisions and the minor ones, all will be scrutinized by those who are looking for "faults" in you, their local Christian example. If we are to attract people to Christ, our lifestyle needs to be as pure as possible. In our information-based society, knowing the information that others know places us at an advantage. We can, through knowledge, show others the follies of the world. We can compare them to the truths of Scripture, and we show them how Christ's love can truly transform their lives.

CHAPTER NINE
Sexual Problems and Issues

The chronicle of Cori's life documents the sexual problems in society over the past 30 years. The year was 1957. Cori was conceived out of wedlock, after an Elvis rock-and-roll concert. Her mother had been married previously and wasn't interested in getting married again, just in having sex.

The year was 1967. At age 10, Cori was awakened from a sound sleep by her 15-year-old brother and two friends who stripped and molested her. Her screams did not deter their abuse, nor were they heard by her mother who was out on a date and had not yet returned home. Cori's recurrent nightmares will be of this episode — the humiliation, the pain and the fear.

The year was 1977. Cori was 20. She was attending a large state university and resided in the front lines, ideologically and personally, of the women's liberation movement. She was especially concerned about the issue of abortion. Accidental pregnancy had led her to have an abortion six months earlier and she wanted to preserve that right for herself and for others.

The year was 1987. Cori, now 30, is married with three children. She became a born-again believer six years ago while watching television as she contemplated suicide with a pistol aimed at her head.

Now she is actively involved with a local pro-life group, marching as often as possible at the local abortion clinic.

Her testimony of conversion has won many young girls to Christ, saving their souls and their precious babies.

Though Cori is now saved, she still suffers from low self-esteem, occasional bouts of depression, panic attacks during her sleep and from marital problems. She is a victim, as are many others, doomed to a lifetime of heartache, all because of sexual problems, rape, premarital sex, abortion and their psychological manifestations.

There are so many stories, so many patients I've dealt with whose lives have been damaged by a sexual incident, a sexual problem or a sexual issue. I've seen the uncontrollable lust created by pornography, the teen woman crushed by her pregnancy and abortion, the young man who is torn between a male and female lover, the woman who was raped. Each represents the sin permitted in our society and the promiscuity present in the church.

How can we stop this emotional and physical carnage? How can we help repair the broken lives of the many victims?

Two answers come to mind, concepts I often use in medical practice. The first is protection, keeping the person from getting the disease or from becoming involved in an accident. Just as we use seatbelts to protect us from injury, we use exercise, rest and nourishment to protect ourselves from illness.

Plague in Our Midst

The second is restoration, allowing the body to heal through care, exercise and discipline until the injured part is again normal. The rehabilitation process restores strength to an injured leg, speech to a damaged brain and lung capacity to infected lungs. The same is true for the sexual problems and issues we all face.

As parents, we are called to protect our children from the enticement that sexual promiscuity offers. We can do this by giving them a scriptural education in attitudes and values. We can also do this by giving them reasons and methods to remain abstinent.

As Christians, we are called to restore, in love, a fallen brother, a wounded sister, a sin-devastated non-believer. The restoration process is a long, slow, arduous task, one that is modeled by the ministry of the Lord Jesus.

We can be used to protect our children and restore others to health when we become prepared servants. Knowledge about these sexual problems and issues gives us a platform from which to minister. Upon knowledge we heap our caring ministry to the broken hearts and devastated spirits. Upon our caring, we share Christ and His power to transform lives.

We will begin with our platform of knowledge, basic information about a number of these problems and issues.

PORNOGRAPHY

Webster defines pornography as "writings, pictures, etc. intended primarily to arouse sexually." The two Greek words that form the root of the word are *porne*, the word for prostitute, plus *graphein*, the word for writing. Webster has in this short definition defined the advertising industry, prime-time and afternoon television programming and many novels, magazines and much popular music. Sexual enticement isn't limited to "pornographic" magazines and movies that show intimate sex by unclothed actors.

Sexual sin through pornography comes in varying degrees

of severity from enticing expressions, postures or clothing to acts of violence, crime and beastiality along with intercourse. As previously described, advertisements associate sexually suggestive facial expressions, posturing and style of dress with a given product to promote an "exciting feeling" so that product will be chosen in the market place. These types of pictures are not usually classified as pornography, but they fill the definition precisely because they use sexual arousal to produce desire for a product.

Initially, soft-core pornography depicted dressed, partially dressed or nude women in alluring poses; but now it encompasses exposure of genitals, couples in the act of intercourse, beatings and other deviant forms of sexual foreplay. Hard-core pornography has also degenerated into showing it all at any time with anyone or anything in incidents of rape, incest, child molestation, murder, bestiality, etc.

Pornography is both a symptom and a cause of our present sexual "state of the union." The pornography magazines emphatically state that viewing their explicitly sexual material satisfies sexual needs, does not create increased desire and does not lead to an urge to view more and more decadent sexuality.

Objective social scientists, however, document that pornography users develop a need to "graduate" to more revealing pictures, seductive language and violent or bizzare forms of intercourse.

The market supposedly dictates to the publishers the type of material people want. But as with any sinful appetite, the more that is consumed, the more that is desired. Those who start using pornography to satisfy sexual urges find pornography available and easy to find. Lesser forms of stimulation do nothing to satisfy their sexual desires. They crave violent and bizarre forms of sexual activity to elicit sufficient arousal. Child pornography, bestiality and sex associated with bondage, rape, and murder are the ultimate fantasies of their sin-ravaged minds.

Plague in Our Midst

Society is damaged indirectly by pornography, through the changed attitudes, hearts and minds of the individuals who have given in to this temptation. Society is damaged directly by the liberalization of sexual attitudes and by the probable increase in sex crimes associated with this addictive pattern. Pornography is often found in the possession of a sex offender or at the scene of a violent sex crime.

Pornography, as with all sexual dysfunction, starts as an individual problem with its own set of causes. Then it becomes a familial and then a societal problem as it grows.

Repeated succumbing to the temptation to view and be excited creates an increased appetite, a psychological addiction, that can grow with each usage.

Larry is a sad example.

Pornography was always around his house — on the coffee table, in the bedroom and in his father's office downstairs. He was allowed to view it at any time and use it to impress his friends. At age nine, he learned to use pornography for self-stimulation. In high school, he spent half of his paycheck on erotic, "hard-core" magazines and pictures through the mail. He was voted the "sex-master" of his fraternity house because of his pornographic connections and his collection of films and videos. His addiction to more violent forms of sexuality continued to grow through college.

His education ended during his senior year when he was accused and convicted of raping, beating and almost killing a college co-ed while he was acting out a popular, pornographic sexual fantasy.

Some sexologists claim that pornography fulfills the need for sex and that it allows the user to put away "hurtful" relationships with members of the opposite sex. Many of these same social scientists forget that you can get caught in an ever-increasing spiral of increasing sexual desire.

Other reasons to use pornography reach into the psychologic nature and needs of an individual. A husband whose sexual needs are not being met by his wife because the wife fears pregnancy may feel justified in viewing pornography to satisfy his desire. A young teen who hears stories from friends about sexual exploits may be curious about how it works and what sex is all about. A lonely widower who's too afraid to think about remarriage may use pornography to meet an unfulfilled sex drive.

Lonely and hurting people who have great unfulfilled needs for affection, love and warmth may use pornography. These people have emotional needs like each of us. Yet these are the ones who become trapped by the addictive self-stimulation while using pornography. Their basic desire for affection drives some into sinful habits, and this solitary fact should make us more willing to urgently reach-out to these lonely people as Christ reached out to us.

HELPING AN ADDICT

Pastors, families, and friends may have a loved one who has become addicted to using some form of pornography and often has little idea on how to deal with the problem. I would like to offer some simple suggestions on helping an addict.

Not starting to use pornography, not filling the eyes and minds with its anti-scriptural philosophies, is the best treatment. But using pornography is like any bad habit, where the individual must first admit that a problem exists and that he or she is willing to deal with the problem.

Changing behavior in an addictive situation begins with determining the extent of the problem. What materials are used, how often are they used and does viewing precede or accompany a sexual act such as masturbation? All forms of pornorgraphy, from explicit magazines to "swim suit issues," need to be taken away. A careful search for hidden "fixes" must be part of the house and mind cleaning.

Being available to the person when an uncontrollable

Plague in Our Midst

craving comes on him, to discuss and encourage the person to try non-sexual, alternative activities, is beneficial. The encouragment and conversation with a spiritual brother can be a blessed distraction. Physical exercise stimulates adrenalin production and provides a very healthy substitute for pornographic stimulation.

Standing in prayer for your addicted friend can provide the accountability and spiritual encouragment needed to shun the appetite. You may want to tell him: "Satan is before the throne of God every day, accusing you of your slavery to your sex habit. I will promise to pray for you daily until your habit is under control. Remember, you have the most important person already praying for you; the Lord Jesus."

If a serious addiction is present and your friend becomes violent or extremely angry, don't try to to help by yourself. You could be seriously hurt. Always seek professional help for the victim and for yourself if needed.

Consistent encouragement, goal setting and repeated counseling are all helpful. Ridding the mind of the abnormal sexual thoughts pornography promotes is a slow process. A solid program of Bible study and prayer will help renew spiritual strength that is depleted by succumbing to sexual temptation.

TEEN PREGNANCY AND ABORTION

Teen pregnancies became an ever-increasing problem during the "free sex" ideologies of the late '60s, '70s and '80s. Most teens, however, do not have the emotional capacity to understand the responsibility associated with intercourse, family or work. Yet their eyes are being opened to sexual "truth" in public school "how to do it" courses. There is little connection between intercourse, the reality of pregnancy and the need for protection with contraceptives in these immature minds.

Presently, the teen pregnancy problem affects one out of four teen women.

Studies of sexuality within the teenage group suggest

that about 50 percent of the women are partaking in sexual relationships and 50 percent of those who partake are getting pregnant. The odds are rather bleak.

Why do these young people have sexual intercourse, protected with contraceptives or not? Many feel peer pressure to "do it" because the group thinks it's "cool." Some very immature teens don't know better. They're curious about their bodily changes and susceptible when a more mature teen wants to show them how. Resisting the strong hormonal urges that are present is too much for some teens. The movies which cater to teens, the magazines and the advertisements all promote "promiscuous" sexuality without the use of contraceptives. It is obvious what the results will be.

Poor family situations may foster rebellion in a teen child, and having sexual relations is one expression of rebellion. Persistent distrust, lack of communication, arguing between teens and parents may frustrate a teen into open rebellion with drug usage, disregard for rules, poor school performance and sexual relations. When a teen cannot find the emotional support, love, encouragement from parents and family, he or she may seek a "love" relationship with another by offering themselves sexually. These immature relationships are short-lived and usually disintegrate with the beginning of pregnancy.

One of the saddest situations I've seen in our society is a teen whose love needs are not met by her parents. She then prostitutes herself for the love her boyfriend promises her or for the love she will receive from her new child. This immature solution to having her needs met results in more disappointment when the boyfriend leaves and no one is there to support her during her pregnancy. When the baby is born more disappointment follows because the infant cannot reurn her love for many, many months. As with other areas of sexual dysfunction, the lack of love by parents or family leads to severe personal and emotional problems in the young mother and her children.

Plague in Our Midst

The rise in teen pregnancies has become one major factor in the epidemic increase in the utilization of abortion clinics. Abortion in the '60s and early '70s became the battle cry for feminists who wanted "freedom" from the responsibility of pregnancy. The surgical procedure was supposed to protect mothers from medical problems during pregnancy; but when the Supreme Court made abortion legal in 1973, the operation quickly became one of the easiest methods of "birth control."

Money and the continued increase in teen pregnancies kept the abortion mills growing and thriving. Public monies were given to large "family planning" groups to pay for the abortions of "poor women." Instantly the profit of providing abortion services attracted physicians who saw the huge profit associated with performing large numbers of abortions in an "assembly-line" set-up. Many obstetricians gave up delivering babies to do the much more lucrative abortion procedure.

Advances since 1973 in the technologies surrounding maternal care, premature infant care, and ultrasound diagnosis have caused serious questioning about the ethical basis of abortion even in secular circles. Most medical problems during pregnancy cause no permanent damage or discomfort for the mother. Far less than one percent of all abortions are done to save the life of the mother. Premature babies can now survive outside of the womb from week 21 of the 40 weeks. Ultrasound has consistently shown the humanity of the child in utero who sucks his thumb, stretches, yawns, hiccups, has fingers, toes, and looks like a baby. Exam by ultrasound during abortion has demonstrated that the infant reacts to pain as his tiny body is pulled apart by the suction instrument.

A few Christians knew better from the start. Now even non-Christians are beginning to understand the horrors of abortion; the pain and suffering for the child; and the depression, anxiety and emotional problems of the mother.

Until the law is changed, abortion will still be legal and

abortion clinics will still exist. But there are a number of activities that we can support and become involved with in helping to repair the personal and societal damage associated with abortion. Supporting pro-life groups and their many educational, legislative and demonstrating activities will slowly but surely turn the tide toward alternatives to abortion.

Churches and individuals should be aware of the rapidly growing "alternative to abortion" movement that is sweeping the country. Many maternity homes are available at no cost to the pregnant young women, and most of these homes provide counseling and direction in matters of keeping or adopting the new child. Some homes even have their own adoption agency available to help place the child with a suitable family. Many offer counseling services and crisis hot-lines for immediate counseling needs, pregnancy testing, clothing, infant needs, and help with medical expenses when residence programs are not offered.

Supporting these pro-life efforts with your prayers and financial aid can help even if you personally cannot become involved.

The ideology of the "world" promotes sexual promiscuity without responsibility and offers abortion to repair the damage done. We need to protect our own children and restore others by offering the scriptural teachings that can prevent these difficult problems and by offering them the restoring love of Christ.

HOMOSEXUALITY

Homosexuality may be the most misunderstood aspect of sexuality because of wide media publicity and the political activism of practicing homosexuals. Yet it is a gross violation of God's principles governing sexuality and it's an "abomination" before Him.

The "world" spreads the philosophy that homosexuality is a "lifestyle," as normal to the homosexual as marriage is to the average couple. Personality, motivation, occupation,

Plague in Our Midst 149

relationships — all are supposedly normal in a practicing homosexual. Any person who suggests otherwise is labeled a bigot.

This abnormal sexual desire, men for men and women for women, the very basis for homosexual practices, is based in the sin nature. But his sin nature alone does not produce these homosexual tendencies and other psychologic changes are often present that help to explain this turn from heterosexuality. How do we know it is based in the sin nature? Individuals who were homosexuals have been able, through the power of the Holy Spirit, to change their sexual orientation and lead normal family lives.

Homosexuality takes on various forms. Many teens have experienced homosexual touching, affection and masturbation expecially at parties where people are using drugs or alcohol. Seldom do these experiences lead to true homosexual affiliation. Some teens have experienced both heterosexual and homosexual relationships and find them both stimulating and rewarding, but they do not continue homosexual relationships once married. But a few individuals who have developed a severe disdain for the opposite sex because they've experienced broken, hurtful relationships do continue to seek only the love offered by partners of the same sex.

In those who have only homosexual relationships, a wide range of personality traits and psychologic dysfunctions are found. A majority of homosexuals come from emotionally unstable homes or single-parent homes where they developed strong attachments to their mother. Many have a problem dealing with assertiveness and dependence, aggressiveness and passivity. Most homosexual men have few demonstrable traits and few admitted psychological problems. Many promote a macho, "beautiful body" image and claim to be normal. This includes their sinful preference for the same sex.

The family and its dysfunction may be the most common source of "changed preferences" from a sexual standpoint.

During healthy psychosexual development, the child identifies with the parent of the same sex, his or her actions, mannerisms and roles. The male child who develops homosexual orientation strongly identifies with the mother, who often is a very dominating person. Males and the father figure are belittled by the dominant mother and male children learn to hate their maleness. Soon females, like mother, stimulate only non-sexual feelings. Males become the object of romantic love as the developing homosexual male seeks an outlet for sexual gratification.

Female homosexuals, or lesbians, often demonstrate similar psychological trauma during formative stages and tend to come from broken, abusive or alcoholic homes where hatred toward males is common.

As with other areas of sexual dysfunction, the breaking apart of the traditional family in our society is to a large degree responsible for the increase in homosexual individuals and for their emerging claim of "normality." It is impossible to violate God's laws of design for human behavior without suffering the consequences. As the homosexual violates God's design and desire for his life, the human body reacts negatively — as seen in the proliferation of such diseases as AIDS.

CRIMINAL SEXUALITY

A sad commentary on our society and its sinfulness is the rampant increase in criminal sexual behavior, ranging from the production and distribution of child pornography to the actual kidnapping, sexual molestation and murder of children and women. Most who perpetrate these crimes have serious antisocial, psychotic or personality problems; some are caught in demon possession, others in satanic worship.

I want to give you a short description of these criminal behaviors and some understanding of their psychological foundations. This will provide you with a surface knowledge to some very serious, individually complex problems.

Plague in Our Midst

Pedophilia is an abnormal desire for and having sex with young, pre-adolescent children. Persons who seek "love" and attention from children are often very immature psychologically. This stems from a lack of psychosexual development past the pre-school or early school level. Pedophiles may fear adult relationships because they have experienced repeated failures in sexual advances to members of the opposite sex. His violence toward the children he entices may be an expression of the anger the pedophile feels toward himself in hating his own childish behaviors. Exposing his genitals to others, viewing others' sexual relationships and homosexual relationships himself may be a part of the pedophile's behavior profile.

Rape is a violent sexual crime where a man forces sexual intercourse upon a known female companion or an unknown female victim. No one personality or psychological disorder can be identified in those who perpetrate rape; but some common traits, such as anger toward females, an abnormally strong sexual drive and failure with other relationships can be seen. A great increase in the number of rapes has occurred because "date rape" and "girlfriend anger" have become reportable crimes. A female who wishes affection short of intercourse may not be able to stop the sex drive of her male companion and it may result in a form of rape. Girlfriends who get mad at their boyfriends after sexual relations have been known to frequent the emergency rooms of hospitals claiming to have been raped, though they were willing during the act.

Incest is the forced or willing sexual relationship between a parent and a child. Abuse of a daughter by a father usually comes about when marital sexual dysfunction (wife withholding sex from husband) is present, and the wife passively approves of the husband using his own daughters as a sexual outlet. The father may have extreme sexual frustration and takes out some of this anger against the wife by "abusing" the daughter(s) in the family. The young girls do not resist because the father threatens or administers violent punishment. Since the mothers often do not resist or intervene in the incest, and since the daughter fears physical reprisal, the solitary or multiple sexual acts are not discovered until guilt and disgust drive the wife or daughter to seek help.

Exhibitionism — exposing genitals to others — is a non-violent, but often serious psychological problem stemming again from broken or mother-dominant homes. Exposure is a passive way to achieve some sexual gratification and/or to show hatred or anger without forcing sex upon another.

Voyeurism — seeking to view others' sexual experiences — is another means of obtaining sexual excitement vicariously through viewing women undressing or observing couples engaged in sexual relations. Pornography is actually a form of impersonal voyeurism not punishable by law.

Both the male and the female derive their sex drive through the presence of androgen in their blood stream, male hormones coming from the testes and female androgens coming from the adrenal glands. Most sexual criminals demonstrate an excessively elevated sex drive, yet studies of their androgen hormones have not shown consistent hormone elevations. Obviously hormones and sex drive are factors as are personality, psychological dysfunction and emotional factors generated by family problems in the home.

Fortunately, these severe problems are rare and seldom encountered by families or by family physicians. But there is a host of more minor, common sexual problems that are found in many families, including those who profess Christ as Savior. The basis for many of these problems are the very lies that are promoted by the world, those that foster selfish, self-indulgent sexuality and describe sex only by its excitement. Stripping sexuality from its God-given principles defrauds those who are intended to benefit from it.

SEXUAL DYSFUNCTION

Sexuality has presented us many problems, of excess, improper usage, abuse and, possibly the hardest to deal with, the problems of missed expectations.

The "world" presents great expectations for sexual encounters, promising that the more one indulges, the greater the pleasure. Faces and bodies painted to perfection and touched-up to remove all blemishes, all beckon to the viewer enticingly shouting sex gives perfect pleasure, a heaven on earth. Perfect women are supposed to crave after men, and women are promised their knight in shining armor will sweep them to happiness everlasting.

The "world" not only presents what cannot be delivered, but it ruins the joy of sex for many people.

Men who have viewed the perfect bodies in many pornography magazines are disappointed on their wedding night, or soon after when they find one imperfection after another in their mates. Romantic, sexually stimulating novels breed heightened expectations about love-making that seldom can be achieved. Sexual relations become the whole intent, purpose, reason and forte for any relationship and for life itself. Without sex a person may as well wither and dry up.

The world's portrayal of male-female relationships is so blatantly anti-scriptural that most Christians easily see through its stimulating facade and reject these premises for marriage relationships. But these philosophies have so infiltrated the media that it is virtually impossible not to take some of these sexual concepts into the bedroom with us as they are carried in our images and thoughts.

Why are thoughts and images so important in the human sexual response? Much of the male sex drive is stimulated by images, enticing behaviors and phrases, types of clothing, states of undress and the female body. Females are stimulated through thoughts of romantic relationships, devotion, protection, as well as the male body. All of these are thoughts that prepare the individual for physical touching and intercourse. Thoughts can be substituted with previous images and actions seen or described in pornography. Thus, the expectations presented in "worldly" sources can fill our "sexual fantasies" with lustful, sin-filled images.

Our hearts and minds belong to the Lord. But without a renewing in regard to sexual attitudes and a constant battle to close our hearing and understanding to the "sexual propaganda" of the media, we can still be tainted and blemished in our thought lives. Filling our minds with memorized Scripture, praying without ceasing and having the strength to "turn off" the explicit media from entering our homes is the most practical way to deal with the problem.

As I've stated, some sexual dysfunction within the Christian home stems from missed expectations rising from the "world's" influence on our minds. Others stem from misunderstandings, fears, and lack of knowledge about sexual attitudes and function. Although I've discussed the more serious sin-based sexual problems — homosexuality, teen-pregnancy leading to abortion, incest, rape, violent sex and pornographic addiction — many other common sexual problems demonstrate not only the "world's" influence on our attitudes, but also the sovereignty of God and His word.

DYSFUNCTION DUE TO WRONG EXPECTATIONS

The term dysfunction is used to define problems within normal marital sexual function. Dysfunctions are common to both Christian and non-Christian and are often caused by expectations that are not true, that are anti-scriptural and that have grown out of a pleasure-seeking mind-set. As the sexual response is mentally derived, these expectations, right or wrong, make or break a person's sex-life. Wrong expectations create a host of problems that I will try to describe.

MARITAL NEWNESS

New married couples eagerly wait for that magic hour when the wedding is over, the reception food eaten, the gifts opened, the farewells bidden, and the threshold broken — the night when wife gives herself to husband and husband gives himself to wife, a loving sacrifice to each other.

Some bring with them excessive baggage, other sexual mistakes, pornographic images, sex-manual "how to's;" and they forget to empty their bags at the door.

The initial newness of a sexual relationship should be treated as any new relationship. The first stage is to get to know the spouse physically and try to understand any fears and apprehensions the other may have about intercourse or pregnancy. Many couples discuss some of these issues before marriage and are well prepared with birth control. The initial newness to sexual intercourse presents certain problems. Mild pain or discomfort for one or both partners is common. This can be lessened with lubricants or relaxation. Problems with the barrier method chosen may occur, such as with a condom or diaphragm, and getting used to the method used may take multiple attempts. Differences in sexual "threshold" or the time it takes to reach climax may be so wide that patience on the part of one partner is essential for the sexual response of the other. Orgasm should not be the ultimate goal as the "world" would suggest; sharing time and affection with each other is. Growing in the physical relationship is more important to the health of the total relationship than a few seconds of adrenalin rush and autonomic nervous stimulation.

If expectations of great "sexual highs" are brought to the marriage bed, pain and frustration may result.

The high pressure of the "world's" expectation to achieve

sexually and reach orgasm is much different from the scriptural, self-sacrificial, loving and patient approach that is guaranteed to help the marital relationship flourish as promised in Scripture.

SEXUAL FEARS

Few individuals bring a "clean slate" to the marriage bed when the wedding is over. Most bring a potpourri of thoughts and remembrances concerning advice, others' experiences and biases toward sexuality.

Some parents have passed their sexual problems and fears along to their children. One mother was so afraid of sexual intercourse with her abusive husband that she warned her daughter that sex was horrible, painful and a way for men to control women. The daughter then took those fears to her marriage bed and withheld so frequently and for such long intervals that the husband threatened divorce.

Fears range from a fear of pregnancy, labor and pain to lack of orgasm and performance. Many women fear the possibility of birth control failure and the pregnancy that results. A child may have been exposed too early to an actual labor experience, not understanding what was occurring. Mothers may pass on to their daughters the images of a miserable experience with delivery, making the daughter feel guilty for the pain and suffering inflicted and unwilling to go through it herself. Men and women alike fear impotence, lack of orgasm, and inability to please their mate. They fear rejection if a "great" sexual performance is not achieved.

Actually, any fears are based on exaggerated experiences and may be a means of displacing guilt from parent to child or a manipulative means of controlling their child's behavior.

Most fears are based on irrational expectations offered by the many avenues of "worldly" information. If orgasm is the only goal suggested by this self-indulgent information, then fear of not achieving becomes rational. But the proper use of intercourse is to share, sacrifice and build the relationship, not to get "high." Intimate sharing, talking, affection, gentleness and time spent together should be the goal, with the added bonus being orgasm.

These fears should all be put aside if posssible. If not, a thorough discussion about them in an honest and open manner will be a trust-building exercise that will allow each spouse to understand and minister more correctly to the needs of their partner.

IMPOTENCE

Impotence is an inability on the part of the male to maintain or achieve an erection. It makes orgasm impossible and decreases the female sexual response.

As previously discussed, much of the sexual response is dependent upon the thoughts and images that are present before and during sexual relations. The psyche limits and can destroy the normal sexual response causing impotence. Thoughts of work and worries of problems and past accidents during relations will limit the response. Fears about failure, lack of orgasm, pregnancy, etc., will also produce failed erections. Apprehension about sexual intercourse following a heart attack or other physical problem may make sexual intercourse difficult if it is not resolved. Most impotence is caused by emotions taken to the marriage bed, problems that should be worked out long before they affect that relationship.

If a woman's mate experiences impotence, she should not blame herself nor worry about some disease or problem with the husband. Instead, a caring willingness to talk about the problems that might be causing it would be appropriate and would build trust and communication between the couple.

Physical problems can cause impotence and a physician should be consulted if lack of erection continues or if other signs of physical disease, such as diabetes mellitus, are present.

FRIGIDITY

Multiple problems with the female sexual response are labeled by an old-fashioned, descriptive term which poorly describes these problems. Frigidity implies coldness or low temperature, but that never occurs — even with a lack of sexual response. There is a parallel between male impotence and its many psychological causes and the female problem of "frigidity."

Generally, frigidity is similar to impotence in physiological or bodily response. The tissues of the vagina and labia do not become engorged with blood, and the vagina does not secrete mucous with intercourse. This leads to uncomfortable, painful relations that destroy stimulation and climax. Just as with impotence, the major cause is the psychological climate, the job problems, home problems, sexual problems and the personal problems that do not allow sexual thoughts to flourish.

Physical problems can precipitate frigidity in the female as some physical problems can cause impotence. Vaginal infections can create inflammation of the vaginal tissues and lead to painful relations and a poor or absent sexual response. Rashes, uterine infections, bladder infections and other health problems can contribute as well.

Vaginismus, the excessive contraction of the muscle ring at the bottom of the vagina, will lead to painful intercourse and a reduced sex drive. Often the fear of intercourse or pain with intercourse will create tension and muscle contraction in that area. Interestingly, fear of pain causes contraction which increases pain which increases tension which increases muscular contraction, etc. Relaxation exercises, alternating the contraction and relaxation of these vaginal muscles, will help alleviate the source of discomfort. Any other contributing psychological issues should be discussed and soothed if possible.

Frigidity can also be seen as a disease of a male-dominated sexual response, perpetuating past cultural biases against the female sexual response. The "world" puts masculinity into a very narrow box, stating to be a "man" you must be able to have multiple "lovers," have intercourse nightly and be "great" each time. Masculinity is orgasm first — pleasing self and then satisfying the partner.

The female often loses when the male's response is predominant, as stimulation may be slower or as each responds at different times. If the male is satisfied sexually, yet the woman time after time is not, she has little motivation to become psychologically stimulated and she loses out again. Male selfishness in a culture that promotes orgasm is an important reason for poor female response.

Some females are taught by their mother that sex is for the male, and the "good girls" endure it and never have orgasm. These older myths have endured for generations and it has taken the "sexual revolution" to make men and women realize that both, with patience, love, and understanding can have a sexual climax. Christian couples who practice sexual relations for the edification of both individuals have discovered this concept and both benefit. Each achieves climax through patience, and the relationship benefits because both parties are building trust and understanding through their cooperation.

SEXUAL OVER-AGGRESSIVENESS

Most married couples have a difference in their sex drive, men usually being more aggressive than women. Changes occur in the sex drive depending upon tiredness, work and home stress, emotional issues and other areas. Scripture speaks of the best way to handle these natural differences through the unselfish giving of self.

> *"The husband should fulfill his marital duty to his wife, and likewise the wife to her husband. The wife's body does not belong to her alone but also to her husband. In the same way, the husband's body does not belong to him alone but also to his wife." I Corinthians 7:3,4 (NIV)*

Sacrificing when the other is ready is the proper way to handle differences, within reason.

Some males have very aggressive sex drives, requesting from their wives sex almost every night, multiple times in the same night, leading on into the morning hours. This may cause discomfort for the wife, along with tiredness, anger and frustration.

Normal sexual function is what is normal for a given couple, anywhere from 4-5 times per week to once every week, month, or season. Needing sex multiple times after getting home from work, needing it on short notice, in different rooms, all can bring frustration and apprehension and lead to a diminished sexual response. This is not normal and must be dealt with through communication, discipline and counseling if necessary.

An excessive need for sex may be a form of addiction to the sex drive which can, through discipline, be controlled to better suit both partners. An over-aggressive partner raises many fears in the mate, from fear of a physical problem causing this uncontrolled behavior to fear of not satisfying the spouse.

Our sexual appetites can be a blessing, a God-given gift to build unity in love between husband and wife, or they can be controlled by the desires of the flesh. There is only one true way to control those runaway desires — by allowing the Holy Spirit to revive the saints and regenerate the sinners.

CHAPTER 10
Design for Revival

There is no greater trauma to a loving parent than to have a rebellious child who turns from God's ways and causes great pain and hurt to himself. I am always disappointed when a patient decides to forego a treatment, one that could relieve a pain or a problem if taken as prescribed. A responsible department head must shoulder great discouragement when those under his authority make disastrous decisions against his advice. A loving husband is crushed when his wife is enticed by another lover to forsake her first love and join in adultery. A philosopher once said, "People will always disappoint you."

A modern ballad laments that we always hurt the ones we love; and, unfortunately, they are the ones we hurt the most. Could it be that our sexual openness hurts ourselves and God?

Our loving, heavenly Father must look at us with a feeling of great disappointment.

How could children whom He loved so much, stray so far from the teachings and the principles He designed to bless, protect and nurture us? How can these children shun bread and choose a stone instead? There must be no greater disappointment than for God to see His rebellious children continuing to hurt themselves.

Maybe I'm in a privileged position, seeing these sexual problems and issues firsthand. The patients I love, care and pray for, are hurt by their sexual desires. Words have not been created that adequately describe the suffering these people will live with everyday for the rest of their lives. Even if we only turn one person away from sexual sin and a lifetime of regret and pain, the whole effort of writing this book will have been worth the investment.

We, as a church and a society, no longer have the privilege of apathy. We know open sexuality is a serious problem, but we do not appear to have the motivation to seek solutions. If the pain associated with broken lives, destroyed families, painful venereal diseases, jealousy and guilt are not enough to move us to action, then maybe AIDS will.

God has set a ringing alarm clock, a clanging cymbal, a blaring trumpet within our hearing to awaken us from our slumber. The church must be stirred to act, especially with the gravity of this plague in our midst.

The plague of AIDS has the ability to destroy the minds and bodies of those attracted to sin. The plague of the heart, the distorted sexual attitudes within the church, has sapped the strength of the church's witness and credibility.

Are we willing to let our young adults risk the very real danger of dying for a moment of pleasure just because we neglected to teach them sexuality from Scripture? Are we willing to allow our society to be torn apart by the issues of teen pregnancy, adultery, divorce, abortion, venereal disease and pornography?

I cannot continue to sit on the sidelines, allowing the worldly philosophies to control the sexuality of my patients or my children. The lives broken by sexual promiscuity are too much for me to see repeated over and over again. Please allow us, Lord, to be a useful instrument, bringing protection, restoration and salvation to those in need.

GOD'S CALL TO RESTORATION

God loves us so much that He has a wonderful solution for this problem.

Even when the church is compromised by sin within its ranks, God can use His word and His principles to call His flock to repentance and to restore them again to fruitful ministry.

When the Jews, God's chosen children, had just completed the greatest work in their history, building the temple of God, He pointed out to them that sin was present and it needed to be purged.

Solomon had just completed the temple when God appeared and said to him:

"If my people, who are called by my name, will humble themselves and pray and seek my face and turn from their wicked ways, then will I hear from heaven and will forgive their sin and will heal their land." II Chronicles 7:14 (NIV)

God has promised to heal our land if we return to His principles.

Our society is also at the height of its accomplishments. We have booming businesses, fantastic technologies and global powers of destruction. The church has never had a greater outreach to so many millions through the mass media. Yet our sinful, anti-scriptural behaviors keep us from being really useful to God.

He can heal our nation from the scourge of sexual immorality when we are ready to follow His design for personal, family and corporate revival.

It is the church, born-again children of God, who must first be purged of wickedness; then our preaching will be heard by sinners.

PERSONAL REVIVAL

I often laugh to myself as I drive past a country Baptist church that displays the following sign year round; "Revival in Progress." Now I see more clearly.

Our hearts must constantly be prepared for revival, every day, all year long. Children of the living God need to be in close fellowship with their Savior through prayer, meditation and reading. Our hearts need to be controlled by the Holy Spirit so that we are not only burdened for the salvation of others, but we also offer God our true repentance when our sinful ideas slip into actions.

Many believers are not in the habit of daily renewal or revival. We must be reminded of the great joy, the renewed power and the personal spiritual success that follows a heart that is revived and committed to the Savior.

God has given us in II Chronicles 7 a pattern of renewal each of us can use to bring ourselves back into closer fellowship with God.

First, we must humble ourselves, realizing the great power and person of God Almighty, and come unto Him with awe and reverence.

Second, we must pray, consistently, specifically for a heart that is broken and contrite before Him.

Third, we must seek His face, through prayer, meditation and reading of His word, so that we will understand the principles to follow and promote.

Fourth, we must repent of any sinful habits, "worldly" ways, unglorifying behaviors that bring sorrow to the Holy Spirit and damage to our fellowship with God.

Are you prepared for the powerful working of God in your life? If you are serious about revival, watch out. The Holy Spirit may point out weaknesses, problems and relationship

Plague in Our Midst

difficulties in our own lives. He may chastise us and bring us down to a heart-felt humility. Many of us have to go through a purging process before the Lord brings revival. This purge-grow, purge-grow cycle is a pattern seen in people and churches who are yearning for God to intervene in their lives.

Personal revival will come in time to the individual who commits himself to follow God's Word in humility, prayer, seeking and repenting.

The reward of personal revival will be the fruits of the spirit, love, joy, peace, etc. — and a renewed desire to share the gospel and lead others to the Savior. Those around us will benefit from this renewed spirit. It will be a living testimony of God's power to heal and restore.

Before we continue, let me ask you a personal question. Some may be reading this text who have never committed themselves to the Savior, never accepted His free gift of salvation and have remained confused by the causes of these social issues. Let me spend a minute sharing with you God's great plan for your life.

God has offered to you, and to me, the blessed gift of salvation. He has allowed people to make this choice for themselves. Some have refused, choosing to follow the course of pleasure and personal fulfillment through power, money, and sexual immorality. Though most people desire these, no one has found lasting fulfillment through these means. We're always seeking more — more power, more money, more sex. God has given us a choice to decide upon this "jetset" lifestyle or to decide that His ways are better.

Jesus Christ was crucified on a wooden cross to pay the punishment for your sins and mine. He proved that He was given power over sin by being raised from the dead three days later. If we accept Him as our Savior, our personal Savior, we too can be given power over sin, death and everlasting banishment in hell. God will forgive our sin and give us new life, eternal life, in Christ Jesus.

If it is your desire to choose God's better way, you may in

prayer come unto him, humbling yourself, seeking His face, and repenting from the sinful, godless lifestyle you are now leading. Here is an example of how you might pray:

> *"Dear Father, I admit that I have been separated from knowing you because I wanted to go my own way. I now admit that I am a sinner, and I accept Jesus Christ as my personal Savior. I gladly give up those sinful habits I know are bad for me and I repent of these and of seeking my own way. Thank you for saving my soul from banishment to hell, and thank you for the guidance and direction of the Holy Spirit You will give me in my daily life. I covenant to read Your word daily, fellowship with You personally through prayer and join with other believers in worship as often as possible."*

If you prayed this prayer and meant it, congratulations. You are now a child of God Almighty. You may want to start reading the Bible, the Gospel of John, chapter three, then the entire book.

FAMILY REVIVAL

God's design for sexuality blesses the family with children, the fruit of a loving, self-sacrificial relationship. Perversion of this design, the self-serving use of sexual intercourse, creates the exact opposite for the family.

Our families are damaged by wrong ideas. The overemphasis on materialism and the desire for pleasurable self-fulfillment both tear the family from its traditional role as provider and sustainer. Children are plucked from the family, enticed by the world's supply of entertainment, comfort and ideas. The safety, shelter and love provided by parents are no match for the excitement offered by others. Our children are being sold to the highest bidder — those

Plague in Our Midst

Children are then willing to learn the values and principles that are promoted through these enticements, those values that place self above God, our needs above others, pleasure above discipline. Scriptural values are placed aside.

Our familes can be restored and revived by the right ideas. Our being examples of biblical values, our caring and loving our children and our consistently seeking God's desires will fill the hungry hearts of our children. Only through the power of the Holy Spirit and revival of individual hearts will revival of the whole family occur.

We can promote revival in our family the same way we can promote it individually. Our family members must recognize their need for God's direction, for group prayer, or study of God's word and for confession and repentance. Praying for the material, health, emotional and spiritual needs of our family, seeing those prayers answered, and seeking guidance in our family decisions will demonstrate God's sovereign design for the family in action.

Our seeking the face of God as a family, our understanding who He is, what He has done and how we should live will mature all members of the family in their spiritual walk. As we confess our sins against one another, we have a double assurance, first of God's forgiveness of sin and second of the power of the family to support through love.

Spiritually maturing young adults are not likely to be swayed by the "world's" enticing glances when they know they have the love and support of their parents backed by the power of God. As they observe scriptural principals in action, they are more likely to make correct sexual decisions that will bring glory to their Savior and honor to their parents.

Our Christian families can be the place where godly principles and values are taught through consistent role models and daily application of scripture. Or it can be the place where our children merely lay their head and eat their meals, but are trained to live by a worldly code of conduct and to walk its broad streets of influence. The choice to restore our families so they can fulfill God's special and holy purpose begins with us, by His grace.

CORPORATE REVIVAL

Revival starts in the hearts of individuals, and it is kindled through repentance and the diligent prayer of those who are seeking the Holy Spirit's intervention. Revival burns with vigor when believers are inspired to commit themselves anew to the basics of Christianity. These include witnessing, teaching and praying. History has shown that once a church is set ablaze with revival, a town, a region and a whole country can be affected by the Gospel of Christ.

Does revival and widespread commitment to the principles of Scripture result in a changed society? Can sexual sin be put aside by those who desire to follow the Lord Jesus Christ?

God's servant Nehemiah was called out of King Artaxerxe's court to rebuild the walls around Jerusalem. All of the Jews came from towns and villages to settle again in Jerusalem; and, when they had come, Ezra gathered them in the square before the Water Gate and read the law. When the people began to understand the law of God, they wept and mourned for their sins.

Ezra read from the law for eight days, hour after hour.

Mourning turned into joy as God's children committed themselves to follow His laws and commandments. Repenting, they separated themselves from the peoples around them and humbly promised to follow all the commands and principles.

Hearing God's word they humbled themselves, prayed for forgiveness, understood His precepts, repented of their error and became involved in a mighty revival.

Jonah was sent to the Ninevites to preach repentance. After a slight detour, he eventually came to the edge of the huge City of Nineveh. He began preaching "Nineveh's doomsday." From that edge of the city, the news spread so

Plague in Our Midst

rapidly that the whole metropolis was set ablaze with spiritual revival. They believed in God through Jonah. They fasted and put on sackcloth. Humbling themselves, praying for forgiveness and repenting from their sin, they saved their city from God's promised destruction.

An entire culture was spared because of the revival of the Ninevites and their heartfelt repentance of their sin.

Revival was also present in the maturing church at Ephesus, early in Paul's ministry. Paul taught, discussed and lectured for almost two years in that city, where Jews and Greeks alike heard the Gospel of Jesus Christ. Many believed because of the Word. Many others believed because of the miracles that were done in the power of the Holy Spirit. Fear for the Lord led many sorcerers to bring their books and publicly burn them, confessing their evil deeds as well as their new faith in Christ. Fifty thousand drachmas of books and scrolls were burned as a public display of repentance.

Corporate revival has spread the Gospel, the Word of God, in many situations over the past 5,000 years. Nations have turned toward the Lord, cities have been saved as individuals have personally trusted God to change their hearts.

Societies in the past have been revitalized when they have heard, heeded and followed the principles of God. Our society today can be turned from sexual sin through the committed prayers of the saints. God would not have allowed the plague of AIDS to afflict our nation and the world, unless He was ready to minister to the many spiritual needs that will follow.

MINISTERING TO THE NEEDY

Our natural reaction to the grotesque sexual depravity we see openly displayed in public is disgust and repulsion. It becomes too easy, however, for our disgust with sin to become disgust for the sinner. It is easy for Christians to judge others and to provide only "negative answers for their complex problems." Instead, we must follow Christ who gave His life on the cross for the people. We must also learn to love the unlovely even in the depts of their sin.

Sexual sin is born within our own desires when we are drawn away by our own lusts. For reference, see James 1:14-15. Temptation leads to sinful attitudes, thoughts, actions, rationalization for the sin and justification for continuing in sin. We are all tempted, but God is able to supply us the strength to resist any temptation.

As fellow sinners reborn to new life in Christ, we can use the knowledge about sexual sin to confront the world with a better solution for its problems. God's solution for the problems of sexuality is a perfect solution.

MEETING PHYSICAL AND EMOTIONAL NEEDS.

Christ was emphatic when He stated, "When you minister to the least of these, you minister to Me." Many have become victims of their own sinfulness, picking up diseases, being beaten by spouses. Children have been sexually molested by fathers. There are pregnant young women who need shelter, love and care.

The church must join in meeting the physical and emotional needs of those touched by the sexual sins of our nation, if the Gospel is to be received. Ministries have begun the task of providing alternatives to abortion by housing young, unmarried women who have been shunned by their families, and their home churches. Babies born to these unwed mothers need homes, loving families to teach them the principles that can save them from repeating their parents' mistake. Counseling, food, clothing, shelter and other physical needs must be provided so that the church can have the privilege of ministering to their spiritual needs.

Meeting the physical and emotional needs of those in violent homes, victims of sexual abuses, who have contracted "sexually transmitted diseases" and those involved with rape or incestuous relations should be a priority of church

Plague in Our Midst

ministries. Needs of this kind can be met through counseling and seminar programs offered by the church, telephone or personal counseling of those involved, and through housing or places of shelter when situations reach a crisis.

Centers supported by the church can offer a variety of ministries, just as a "crisis-pregnancy center" offers shelter, counseling and physical necessities to teen mothers. These church centers offer the protection, shelter and support that can be given to begin the recovery process. It is when those in need can see the love of Christ in the sacrifice of the laborer and through the Word shared with them.

A greater area of need will be to minister to the emotional and physical needs of those afflicted with the AIDS virus, the opportunistic infections and tumors. Centers where AIDS victims can reside, work productively, be ministered to emotionally and spiritually will be required as the numbers of AIDS-infected persons rise into the millions. Their spiritual renewal will ease the pain and agony of living with the scars of their sin. Only through Christ will they receive the forgiveness that can brighten their outlook, even unto death.

Fundamentalist and evangelical denominations should set up AIDS centers to minister to the many needs of the victims. Just as Christ ministered to those with leprosy, the most dreaded disease of the Roman culture, Christ through the church can minister love, acceptance, and salvation to those with the greatest physical needs today.

MEETING SPIRITUAL NEEDS

Secular counselors become extremely frustrated with clients when their advice seemingly falls on deaf ears. But the power to intervene in sinful habits, the adulterous relationships, the pornographic habits, the addiction to the bizarre forms of sex is available only through the Holy Spirit — and that only through salvation in Christ.

We can debate the issues of diseases associated with promiscuous sexuality until we are blue in the face and yet not change the minds of those sold on excitement through sex. We can warn our secular friends about the emotional fallout, the guilt and anger, when an adulterous relationship is discovered, but will we be able to persuade them to stop seeking other sinful relationships? We can even warn our children of the extreme dangers of contracting AIDS and lose them to the emotional arguments of their peers.

We are powerless to beat sin through our intellect, persuasion, debating, psychological advice. Only Christ's power to regenerate the heart and change the life can defeat sin.

Persons who realize that their sexual habits are sinful often react defensively. Once on the defensive, they can find an excuse, a rationalization, a justification for any argument against the sin. Only our love shown through the word and deed, can open their defensive, self-indulgent hearts.

Christians should not be ashamed to share with non-Christians the facts about sexual perversion in our society. Knowledge is a powerful and well-respected tool at our disposal to make others aware that promiscuous sexuality is creating severe and dangerous problems for all of us. Once we have gained their attentive ear, we can offer the real solution to sexual problems, namely salvation through Christ and obedience to the scriptural principles of sexuality.

Do we deserve their attention if we are too lazy to understand the world around us? Do we dare preach at them when we are equally sinful before God? Do we dare turn them off to the Gospel with our judgmental airs of self-righteousness, instead of with the love God offers so freely to us?

EPILOGUE

Remember Jay? He is now in the final stages of AIDS.

It has been a few weeks since I heard about his last admission to the hospital. He had been feeling poorly and had a persistent cough for about one month. The chest X-ray showed that infection was present in his lungs. Further tests proved that the infection was due to an opportunistic infection common to AIDS patients, Pneumocystis carinii. After two different antibiotics, the infection finally ended.

The decision was made to place Jay on the new drug, AZT. When he called me two weeks after starting the medication, he was extremely pleased because he had no side effects. But he still knew that the end was just beginning.

When a patient begins to succumb to the numerous opportunistic infections of AIDS, it means that he or she may have a few months to approximately two years to live. The drug AZT does not cure the AIDS virus. It only slows its spread. Thus AZT may prolong Jay's life, but nobody knows how long.

The bad news is that Jay doesn't have long to live.

The good news is that Jay is being helped, physically, emotionally and spiritually.

Through the sorrow, the devastation of learning about Jay, God opened a number of doors for an AIDS ministry. The specifics, the place, who is being ministered to and how must remain quiet to protect the identity of these victims. But God has allowed us to open an AIDS ministry for the innocent victims of this terrible disease.

Other Christian-based AIDS ministries are beginning elsewhere. In a western state, a converted homosexual has started his own ministry. He is known and trusted and he can speak to the needs of homosexual AIDS victims through experience.

This gentleman is visiting AIDS victims, bringing them Scripture, running errands and shopping for them, raising money for clothing and food when their funds are depleted. This man is helping where others will not. The fruits of his love are seen in the men who have given their lives to Christ, many on their death beds. Is it time for you to help, too?

Our families need protection from this deadly situation, through spiritual renewal and the teaching of God's principles for sexuality. Our churches need to be purged of the plague of the heart, repenting and following God's principles for sex within marriage. Our society needs to hear a clear, consistent, credible message from the church — that promiscuity is sin and that abstinence is the only right decision.

It is time that each of us becomes actively involved in understanding God's principles for sexuality.

It is time for us to follow these principles personally.

It is time for us to teach these principles to our children and to lovingly meet people with the Gospel at their point of need. Then and only then will the plague in our midst be ended.